PSYCHOLOGY LIBRARY EDITIONS: SPEECH AND LANGUAGE DISORDERS

Volume 5

SIGNS, SIGNALS AND SYMBOLS

SIGNS, SIGNALS AND SYMBOLS

A Presentation of a British Approach to Speech Pathology and Therapy

Edited by
STELLA E. MASON

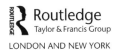

LONDON AND NEW YORK

First published in 1963 by Methuen & Co. Ltd

This edition first published in 2019
by Routledge
2 Park Square, Milton Park, Abingdon, Oxon OX14 4RN

and by Routledge
52 Vanderbilt Avenue, New York, NY 10017

Routledge is an imprint of the Taylor & Francis Group, an informa business

© 1963 The College of Speech Therapists

All rights reserved. No part of this book may be reprinted or reproduced or utilised in any form or by any electronic, mechanical, or other means, now known or hereafter invented, including photocopying and recording, or in any information storage or retrieval system, without permission in writing from the publishers.

Trademark notice: Product or corporate names may be trademarks or registered trademarks, and are used only for identification and explanation without intent to infringe.

British Library Cataloguing in Publication Data
A catalogue record for this book is available from the British Library

ISBN: 978-1-138-34553-9 (Set)
ISBN: 978-0-429-39880-3 (Set) (ebk)
ISBN: 978-1-138-36799-9 (Volume 5) (hbk)
ISBN: 978-0-429-42946-0 (Volume 5) (ebk)

Publisher's Note
The publisher has gone to great lengths to ensure the quality of this reprint but points out that some imperfections in the original copies may be apparent.

Disclaimer
The publisher has made every effort to trace copyright holders and would welcome correspondence from those they have been unable to trace.

SIGNS
SIGNALS AND
SYMBOLS

A PRESENTATION OF
A BRITISH APPROACH TO
SPEECH PATHOLOGY AND THERAPY

EDITED BY
STELLA E. MASON

LONDON
METHUEN & CO LTD
36 ESSEX STREET · WC2

First published 1963
© *1963 The College of Speech Therapists*
Printed in Great Britain by
Richard Clay & Co. Ltd, Bungay, Suffolk
Catalogue No. 2/2596/10

CONTENTS

	INTRODUCTION	*page* ix
1	LANGUAGE, LIFE AND LITERATURE *The Right Reverend the Lord Bishop of Birmingham, J. L. Wilson*	1
2	THE PLACE OF "SPEECH THERAPY" AMONG THE SCIENCES *L. Stein*	7
3	SIGNS AND SIGNALS *W. Haas*	20
4	LINGUISTICS AND SPEECH PATHOLOGY *J. L. M. Trim*	33
5	HISTORICAL LINGUISTICS *Alan S. C. Ross*	44
6	THE QUANTUM OF LANGUAGE *G. Patrick Meredith*	50
7	CODING AND DECODING IN SPEECH *D. B. Fry*	65
8	AIDS TO DIAGNOSIS AND THERAPY *John R. Brook*	83
9	EVALUATING THE NATURE AND DEGREE OF DEFECTS AND DISORDERS OF VOICE, SPEECH AND LANGUAGE *Joan H. van Thal*	87
10	SIGN-POSTS IN DIAGNOSIS *C. H. Aldridge*	93
11	THE SUPPRESSION OF THE SIGNAL *Peggy Carter*	101

CONTENTS

12 BREAKDOWN IN COMMUNICATION IN A NINE-YEAR-OLD BOY *M. J. L. Ellis* — 109

13 CHILDREN'S DRAWINGS—THEIR VALUE IN THERAPY *Joan Pollitt* — 117

14 INFORMATIVE AND MANIPULATIVE SIGNS AND SIGNALS IN LANGUAGE DISORDER *Stella E. Mason* — 131

15 THE DATA UNDERLYING THE CONCEPT OF DYSLALIA *R. E. Simms* — 141

16 ANALYSIS OF THE LINGUISTIC DATA OF DYSLALIA *L. M. Hartley* — 152

17 TOWARDS A NEW CONCEPT OF DYSLALIA *P. A. E. Grady* — 159

18 CLUES IN APHASIA *Joyce L. Wilkins* — 166

19 THE ASSESSMENT OF DEFECTIVE SPEECH IN AN ADULT *D. B. Fitch* — 175

20 A CRITICAL INVESTIGATION INTO THE PROBLEM OF DYSARTHRIA *Lyn P. Parker* — 183

21 A PILOT SCHEME FOR SPEECH THERAPY IN TRAINING CENTRES *Olivé Duffie* — 195

22 SPEECH THERAPY WITH BACKWARD CHILDREN *Catherine E. Renfrew* — 201

23 SOME PROBLEMS FACING THE ADULT WITH PROGRESSIVE DEAFNESS, AND LIPREADING *D. F. Collins* — 205

INDEX — 209

ACKNOWLEDGEMENTS

Special thanks are due to the Oxford University Press for permission to reproduce a passage from A. Gardiner's Egyptian Grammar.

The illustrations in Chapter 15 are redrawn by kind permission of the publishers Raben & Sjögren.

INTRODUCTION

Reference to speech disorders and their treatment can be found in many writings ever since antiquity, but the pathology and therapy of speech, language and voice disorders as an organized body of knowledge has been in existence for only a few decades.

Treatment, which consists in the testing of predictions contained in a hypothesis, relies on accurate diagnosis. It may be argued that the validity of a curative method lies in "success", but this claim must be refuted since in many cases the affliction appears to be alleviated although the curative measure has not altered it but has merely obliterated one of its symptoms; for instance, morphia administered in a case of appendicitis relieves the pain but does not cure the appendicitis. Similarly, the removal of consequential habits in a stammer by no means abolishes the deep-lying factors that are at work in the stammerer's personality. Everyone who possesses the faculty of hearing knows if a person has a stammer, lisp or nasal speech, but not everyone understands the nature of the abnormality or the elements underlying this abnormality; to say that a person stammers is a comment, it is not a diagnosis. Determining how the elements are structured in a given speech or language disorder, thereby forming a hypothesis and making a diagnosis on which therapeutic procedure may be based, is a responsibility that has in this country been undertaken only, so far, by the members of the profession represented by the College of Speech Therapists. It is desirable to make this point clear, for it still seems to many lay and professional people that it is the function of the "speech therapist" merely to "correct" speech that is faulty, "teach" language where it is deficient and perhaps to function on prescription from the physician, the surgeon or the psychiatrist.

Therapists have to solve practical problems; their main concern is to help people overcome their difficulties or impediments in the

INTRODUCTION

use of language. To study adequately any breakdown in communication, it is necessary first to understand the nature and structure of the particular mode of communication that has ceased or not begun to function and, in presenting findings, to adopt a system of investigation amenable to analysis. Information should be given of the results of observation in unambiguous terms, for in no other way is it possible for other inquirers to check up on assertions which, when they are first made, are only believed to be true and await verification. Terms of reference are required in order that workers within a profession and – ideally – allied professions may understand one another. To argue that technical terms should not be used because their meaning is unknown to those outside the profession is to argue that a doctor should use, perhaps, the word "cancer" rather than "carcinoma" for the same reason. Translation into the vernacular is necessary in all professions when the occasion requires it. Yet information of the results of observations cannot be given solely by use of the vernacular, for no two different semantic units are completely identical.

"Some hold translations not unlike to be
The wrong side of a Turkey tapestry." [1]

As an example, the everyday use of the term "word" is not accurate or precise enough for purposes of scientific investigation, for a word is an arbitrary, not a fixed, segment of utterance (should "inasmuch" be regarded as one word or three?) and sentences, that is, communicative utterances of some length, are not merely combinations of single sounds.

This book is based on papers read by members and their guests at a National Conference of the College of Speech Therapists held in Birmingham in 1961. The organizers agreed to adopt as the theme of the Conference the principal concept of Communication Theory, according to which language can be regarded as a system of Signs, Signals and Symbols. To justify and elaborate this idea, eminent workers in the fields of linguistic theory and psychology were invited to confer with the delegates on the application of these principles, thereby sharing with members of the College the outcome of their learning and experience.

[1] James Howell (1645–55) Letters, Book 1, 6

INTRODUCTION

Recognition was given to the Conference by the Lord Mayor of Birmingham, Alderman Eric E. Mole, and great honour was given to the profession by The Right Reverend the Lord Bishop of Birmingham, J. L. Wilson, who gave the Inaugural Address and has most graciously allowed a shortened version of his speech to be published here. The guest speakers whose papers are included in this book, and to whom I wish to express our grateful thanks, are Professor D. B. Fry, PH.D (London University), Mr W. Haas, M.A. (Manchester University), Professor G. P. Meredith, M.SC., M.ED., PH.D., F.B.PS.S. (Leeds University), Professor A. S. C. Ross, M.A. (Birmingham University) and Mr J. L. M. Trim, M.A. (Cambridge University). I am glad to have the opportunity of acknowledging my gratitude for the generous cooperation of the publishers, Messrs Methuen and Co.

Although the contents of this book may fairly be said to represent a British approach to speech and language pathology and therapy, it makes no claim to be a textbook. Those who undertake the treatment of speech and language disorder must necessarily cover a wide area, and it was not the intention to make the Conference an occasion for a comprehensive survey of speech therapy nor to adhere rigidly to the original interpretation of the theme contained in the title. A collection of papers written by various authors generally results in the expression of differing opinions. Needless to say, it was hoped that all contributors would approach the problem with all the meticulous care and humility of scientific inquirers, for until such time as all those who administer treatment do so, there will continue to be conflicting ideas on methods of treatment that must inevitably lead to disappointment and distress on the part of both the therapist and the patient.

Martinet, writing about modern linguistics, said that people do not like to be disturbed. Change is a disturbance and progress results in change; if change gives rise to anxiety this in its turn may lead to hostility. It would then be hardly surprising if some of the new and different notions expressed in this book produced hostility as a first reaction. Yet it is said that memory is a fond deceiver and it is not unknown for ideas that produce adverse criticism when first put forward to be claimed later by others as their original thoughts. "Queer thing the mind. Read those Viennese fellows and you'll see

INTRODUCTION

one can't be too careful with it."[1] Taking heed of this warning and before memory fades or deceives, I wish to place on record that although the work involved in the organisation of the Conference was done by a small committee, to the loyal members of which I offer my grateful thanks, its concept was the inspiration of Dr Leopold Stein. It was he who put forward the idea for the theme and for the publication of the papers in this form, he who gave such generous advice to many of the less experienced contributors and assistance in countless other ways. It was in the knowledge that I could call on his help and reap the benefits of his wisdom and breadth of vision that I agreed to take on the exacting responsibilities involved in the organization of the Conference and the editing of this book. Our debt to Dr Stein is one that is difficult to repay.

Stella E. Mason

Birmingham 16

---

[1] Michael Innes (1944) *The Weight of the Evidence*, London, Gollancz

I

THE BISHOP OF BIRMINGHAM
(Dr J. L. Wilson, C.M.G.)

Language, Life and Literature

An inaugural lecture ought really to be given by one who is technically competent to survey the whole field of this conference. That, alas, I cannot do. But I hope I shall at least say enough to show how importantly I regard its work. Perhaps some of my thoughts may be echoed, or even controverted, in its lectures and discussions.

I want, however, to begin by saying something about therapy and religion because I am convinced of its relevance to the profession of speech therapy and work in allied fields.

The therapeutic value of religion depends entirely upon its ability to contribute to the relief of the mental anguish and physical suffering that accompany physical disease, mental distress and social maladjustment.

In therapeutics we have two great groups of remedies. One is devoted to the amelioration of symptoms and is designed to relieve the patient's suffering, thus indirectly contributing to a hopeful state of mind and an improvement in morale. The other is aimed more directly at the removal of the causes of the disease and is, of course, by far the more efficient method of treatment.

When we examine religion as a therapeutic agent we find that almost any form of religious belief – faith in a Supreme Being, confidence in the supernatural – seems to possess therapeutic value when looked at from the symptomatic standpoint; that is, it helps the sufferer temporarily by enabling him to minimize his sufferings and externalize his thinking. Not all religious beliefs aim at the cause of sickness and suffering, and therefore they are not fundamentally true therapeutic agents in the real and curative sense.

In organic disease we must recognize that religion is not a curative therapeutic agent; it can only serve as a palliative. But in the functional diseases religion serves a great purpose. It augments morale: it sometimes lessens suffering: it promotes hope and courage: it contributes to that determination that is a part of the cure of every sick person who recovers. But it is in the domain of mental and nervous disorders, the field of mental medicine, that religion exerts such a tremendous influence, and this, after all, constitutes the great bulk of human sickness and distress. I have no way of proving it, but nevertheless I firmly believe that apart from surgical disorders, contagious diseases and accidents, nine tenths of the sickness and suffering that come to a doctor is directly or indirectly the result of the mental state and nervous attitude of the patient. They belong to the domain of mental medicine, and it is in this realm that religion functions as the master mind-cure.

The real cause of most human suffering and unhappiness is fear – that fundamental emotion associated with the instinct of flight that so valuably served our primitive ancestors as a survival-reaction, but which has, under the conditions of modern civilization, come to be associated with the modern defence-reaction of civilized races, the flight from reality. Fear is now largely used by the so-called subconscious mind to conjure up a thousand alibis, camouflages and other defence-reactions to help unconscious cowards flee from reality, dodge difficulty and get out of doing disagreeable things.

Religion becomes a real and basic cure for the disorder of fear when it is a religion that inspires faith. Faith is the only known cure for fear, and religious faith is the master faith-cure. No other form of faith can sweep through the mind and annihilate fear with such certainty and power as religious faith. Religion is one of the basic human emotions and, with its associated group of feelings and sentiments, is able, in the case of the average human being, to dominate the entire personality, and even to control those almost equally powerful emotions, the desires for significance and sex.

It is in this sense that Christianity becomes one of the most powerful of known therapeutic agents. The Christian religion is therapeutically and psychologically sound – at least the teachings of Jesus are. They carry with them the therapeutic attitude of faith triumphing over fear. They beckon struggling mortals to self-confidence and superb courage in meeting all the harassments of life. Universal acceptance of the teachings of Jesus would serve to wipe out the whole disease-category of those disorders resulting from social vice, intemperance and drug habits.

Religion is also a wonderfully efficient antidote for monotony. One of the greatest causes of monotony is this machine age. The tendency to specialization of labour is increasingly robbing the individual artisan of opportunity for self-expression. Religion enables us to live in two worlds, often in many worlds simultaneously, and is going to prove a valuable antidote for social unrest, economic dissatisfaction and increasing psychic disquietude.

Religion stimulates the speculative faculties and broadens the horizon of the imagination. Man is naturally an adventurer. Civilization is gradually lessening man's opportunity for experiment and adventure, but religion – at least, a true vision of the teachings of Christ – opens before man vistas of universal dimensions and transcendant grandeur. In imagination the depressed soul looks at a universe he hopes subsequently to journey through as a translated spirit-personality. A stimulating religion of this sort satisfies curiosity and does something to gratify our craving for adventure.

The practice of prayer can be either a means of augmenting one's mental suffering or a powerful curative agent. When prayer grows out of forebodings of doom to come, then it certainly adds to human misery. When one prays over some trifling besetment it only serves, by auto-suggestion, to fasten the habit upon the praying soul more securely. But when prayer is a real spiritual communion, a service of praise and thanksgiving; when prayer contains more of worship, in that it ceases to ask anything for the one who prays; when it comes to be an expression of gratitude and praise to the Creator for what his creature envisages the Creator to be – then prayer becomes a marvellous dual therapeutic agent. It has a sedative effect, bringing sleep to troubled minds and rest to distraught souls. It also exerts a tonic effect in that it spurs the indolent to action and urges the doubting and fearful forward to new conquests and greater victories.

Religion is an antidote for narrow introspection. It provides a universal outlook. An egocentric religion has little permanent therapeutic value. Jesus taught a religion that reaches out even to the "many mansions". Philosophy is entertaining, diverting and has therapeutic value. But nothing else has the power or influence possessed by faith in a personal Deity. Christianity, through the Master, provides a real and living way between the creature and the Creator.

Of the five great world religions, Christianity does most to meet the demands of a therapeutic agent. It lessens fear and self-contemplation, it stimulates spiritual vision and enlarges the intellectual horizon. It makes possible a philosophy that is consistent with history, science and civilization, and these three things constitute the yardstick whereby we should measure any religion to ascertain its medical and social therapeutic value.

Both the Old and New Testaments link the idea of health with religion. All through the Old Testament the effect of fear upon both happiness and health was coming into recognition. "Fear not" is the perpetual injunction of the New Testament. Many times the Master said to the sick, "Thy faith hath made thee whole". No more powerful medicine can be given the victim of an anxiety-neurosis than the sustenance that is to be found in the belief of such promises as "casting all your care upon Him; for He careth for you". The whole question of religion as a therapeutic agent is summed up by St John, who said: "There is no fear in love; but perfect love casteth out fear: because fear hath torment".

I would, then, most emphatically affirm that religion is a therapeutic agent; that all religions are of value in alleviating symptoms. I would go further and say that the Jewish and more especially the Christian religions are basically curative in that they strike at the root of most mental disorders – they substitute faith for fear. I would go further still and say that Christianity is the master mind-cure, the superlative therapeutic agent, designed to relieve those mental attitudes of fear, doubt, unrest, dissatisfaction, monotony and loneliness. And when I make this statement I refer to Christianity not as it has been misrepresented by scores of its mediaeval and even of its modern advocates, but as it was proclaimed two thousand years ago, according to the records, by Jesus of Nazareth.

I make no apology for speaking of my faith in this matter, for as a seeker after truth I am firmly convinced that *life* – life now and life eternal – can be found in the knowledge of Jesus and His teaching. It could be and in many cases *is* the most valuable aid to therapy.

I have spent most of my time presenting my views on therapy and religion because I deem it important. What about speech and language?

Unless those who have something valuable to say in the sphere of religion and politics learn how to speak their words clearly, lucidly and persuasively, we shall be at the mercy of the smooth-tongued emotional evangelist and the rabble-rouser. For the tongue, if not mightier than the sword, is certainly mightier than the written word in its *immediate* appeal. How important then is this subject of speech, not merely for those who suffer handicaps and inhibitions, but for all those who in any way have the duty of communication, such as teachers, preachers, readers and all those who are called to speak in public.

It is falsely and tacitly assumed that the faculty of speech is a sort of instrument which, by some intuitive power, may be played upon with varying degree of skill by the most uninstructed amateur. In no other art would anyone, without the boldest effrontery, dare to inflict himself upon an audience until he had undergone some course of training; but in the art of public speaking the almost universal opinion is, by implication, that the extemporaneous speaker is the product of some accidental growth.

Such a notion is contrary to the opinions and practice of both ancient and modern orators. In ancient Greece and Rome men were orators not by nature or accident, but became such by education and training. Cicero said that speakers are made, not born. It is true that a man must be born with certain qualities without which true oratory would be impossible. These, however, in some degree all men possess. Yet not even the possession of these inborn qualities can take the place of judicious and well-directed training. All our powers of mind and body begin in imperfection and need development and expansion. So it is with the power of speech, and the speech therapist has his part to play in this most important task.

I would like to close with two quotations about literature. The first is from the Preface to James Sutherland's *The Oxford Book of English Talk*:

"Nothing, surely, can bring us closer to the day-to-day life of earlier generations than the voices of those men and women who once lived in that present which is now the past [he writes]. We can hear them speak to each other, quarrelling, grumbling, gossiping, bullying, prevaricating, merry and sad, drunk and sober, eloquent and inarticulate. What we listen to then is the living voice – 'at once far-off and near'."

My second quotation is from Henry Ward Beecher. He writes:

"Part of our work is to teach the body to serve the soul; and in this work the education of the voice is an important part. The human voice is like an orchestra. It ranges high up, and can shriek betimes like the scream of an eagle or it is low as a lion's tone; and at every intermediate point is some peculiar quality. It has in it the mother's whisper and the father's command. It has in it warning and alarm. It has in it sweetness. It is full of mirth and full of gaiety. It glitters (tho' it is not seen) with all its sparkling fancies . . . and men listen to it through the long hour, wondering that it is so short, and quite unaware that they have been bewitched out of their weariness by the charm of a voice, not artificial, not pre-arranged in the man's thought, but by assiduous training made to be in his highest nature. Such a voice answers to the soul."

2

L. STEIN, London

The Place of "Speech Therapy" among the Sciences

The implications of the theme Signs, Signals and Symbols, as well as those of the title of this paper, cannot be considered without first looking back at the "prehistory" of The College of Speech Therapists.

At a time when speech therapy was represented by two corporate bodies I advocated in a paper published as far back as 1942 that a college should be founded. My reason for doing so, and for suggesting the word college rather than society, association or any other name, was that in current usage a college is a possibly chartered corporation of scholars who abide by certain rules, a body whose stature is comparable to that of a university. The purpose of our college, as set out in its articles, is "to promote the Art and Science of Speech Therapy and its interrelation with any branches of knowledge or professions related thereto".

The idea of a college is opposed to that of an ancillary body. "Ancillary" comes from Latin *ancilla* "servant girl, handmaiden", literally "the one who bustles about".

The title of this paper asserts that there are entities called sciences and that one of them is speech therapy. If it is a science, why call it therapy? Other sciences on which treatment is based are usually referred to by a word compounded with the suffix *-logy*, such as laryngology, dermatology. We do not speak of laryngotherapy. If it is our claim that we do not treat symptoms but that we try to find and handle the factors responsible for the symptoms, then speech therapy is a misnomer. What we must avoid is the confusion between what a thing is and what it is recognized or labelled as.

In order to know what the subject of one's inquiry "is" the following scientific procedures are employed:

1. Adequate observation.
2. Proper description.
3. Arrangement of the data in a suitable space-time framework.

From these three procedures assumptions are derived regarding the "true" state of affairs and what the subject matter "is".

4. Experimentation that is based on prediction, making it possible to verify the assumptions.

Let me illustrate briefly: someone not familiar with electricity has observed that light comes on when the lever of a thing, labelled switch and described minutely, is turned up or down. He then assumes that he knows how light is created. (This is comparable to the assumption that "tension" creates stammer!) If he is wise enough not to take anything for granted he will finish his investigation with procedure four. To fix a switch on the wall and operate it will show him that his assumption regarding the nature of light is wrong. If he proceeds again under the guidance of the rules I have mentioned, he will ultimately gain true knowledge of the essence of electric light (or, for that matter, of stammering).

To sum up, the scientific inquirer deals with what is empirically given by means of logical operations alternating with observation, description, arrangement, prediction and experimental verification.

These guiding lines are common to *all* sciences. Yet there must be criteria by which we can distinguish one science from another. It is easy enough to state what the subject of our inquiry is. We are concerned with language or "what is being said". So are other workers such as neurologists, psychologists, plastic surgeons or linguists. The members of this profession, if they claim to represent a profession of their own cannot, therefore, content themselves with stating that they follow the general method of scientific inquiry. Rather is it necessary to demonstrate that their approach is distinct and unique inasmuch as it is adapted to the subject, scope and aim of the discipline. In order to prove the claim that they have a profession in its own right, it is necessary to describe the contributions made by other scientists to the knowledge of language, and by contrast to show that our approach leads to a distinctive explication of the phrase "what is being said" with particular emphasis on operational statements.

My exposition of the work of other scientists is necessarily very brief.

Those mainly concerned with language are:

1. Linguists
2. Teachers of languages
3. Psychologists
4. Sociologists
5. Anthropologists
6. Biologists
7. Communication theorists
8. Speech therapists, so called.

(1) The *linguists* can be subdivided into several groups, such as (*a*) phoneticians, (*b*) synchronic linguists, (*c*) diachronic linguists.

(*a*) The phonetician explores the elements of speech and provides the means for observing and describing them (Haas, 1957, 58), either in terms of physiological or articulatory, or in terms of acoustic categories (Ibid., p. 129).

Much too little use has been made by speech therapists of the apparatus devised by the phonetician.

(*b*) The synchronic linguist observes the relations of the elements within a language in order to build a model showing the structure of the linguistic code and to develop a theory of the design of language and of particular languages (Haas, 1954, 55).

(*c*) The diachronic linguist (philologist) looks at language in relation to cultural, social, literary and historical material and traces its features back to those of earlier stages. He can do so because he has developed a special method which has become the standard for other methodologies. One of the procedures is the purposive comparison of features belonging to different levels of time and to different areas of the same level. By this method general trends towards phonological change (an example of this being palatalization) and towards semantic change have been discovered; for instance the word "belief" from "lief" an older form of "love" and kindred with *libido*. Some therapists have taken due notice of this invaluable procedure, but regrettably only few problems of speech therapy have been approached in that manner.

(2) The *teachers of languages* naturally have an interest in the study of languages and their features. Their notions are largely based on those of traditional grammar. They tacitly assume that there are certain norms of talking accepted in particular social settings. These models are not intended to explain the phenomena, but to perpetuate the standards. This implies the assumption of an ideal language which by its nature is perfect, and that only the usage may be at fault.

(3) The *psychologists* of various denominations look upon language as the finished article, as one function of the human mind. Their endeavour is to detect the laws governing the conscious and unconscious motives for linguistic communication, dynamics, perception of and the responses and adjustments to language. The child psychologist pays particular attention to the development of the faculty of language in relation to the growth of other capacities such as thinking, feeling and learning. He is concerned with what the acquisition of language does to the child and the impact of the child on the system of communication he is acquiring (Hockett, 1958). Many psychological investigations of language have unfortunately been marked by failure to take account of the results of linguistic science. Conversely, and equally deplorably, few workers in the field of language are acquainted with the methods of psychological interpretation (Carroll, 1959).

(4) The *sociologist* deals with language or any other activity in connection with the structure of and the interaction between social groups. The sociologist is interested in individuals only insofar as they play different roles according to the group to which they belong at any given time. Take, for instance, the subject of clothing. The garments worn by men and women differ in various national and social groups. Women in Western countries now wear short skirts in everyday life, while in Sumatra and Celibes the exposure of the knee is considered as immodest as it was considered in Europe not so long ago.

It is well to remember the difference between the two closely related, hence often confused concepts of the sociologist, those of social relations and social structure (Lévi-Strauss, 1953, p. 525).

Social relations are given to us through observation while structure is a model built by us. This model has the characteristics of a system of elements, none of which can undergo a change without affecting the others. This makes intelligible all observable facts and enables us to predict reactions if any of the elements are subjected to modification. The sociologist might, perhaps, not only make a study of sartorial customs in various groups but also of the effect on a group if an individual's dress does not conform to the established standard. A number of men attired in swimming trunks on the beach would form one group or system of elements. The same men dressed in black coats, pin-stripe trousers and bowler hats would, from the sociologist's point of view, form another group. If one of the elements in either system undergoes modification a reaction can be predicted. For instance, if one man joins either group wearing black coat, bowler hat and swimming trunks this modified element affects the whole. The sociologist would also note the effect on social groups if language patterns differed from the accepted standards. An illustration of the value of the social structure model in diagnosis and therapy is observable in the reactions of groups to speech and language idiosyncracies and abnormalities. Language varies according to whether one speaks to children or adults, in the drawing room or in the bedroom and so on.

(5) Man and his evolution in all aspects is the subject of *anthropology* inasmuch as it concerns itself with the physical characteristics of human beings as well as with all human activities such as tool making, building, art, customs and beliefs, that is, their culture patterns, of which language is one. The anthropologist also studies the relation between language and other culture patterns. It is he who tells us, for instance, that in the languages of primitive groups rhythmical utterances are frequently used and sanctioned (cf. Lubbock, 1889). It is for us to utilize such observations in the evaluation and treatment of speech disorders, such as stammering and aphasia (Stein, 1942). The study of the evolution, that is, integration of language, is vital to anyone who has had to deal with its dissolution (cf. Jackson, 1958).

(6) The *biologist* studies the needs and drives of living beings and the significance of their behaviour, both innate and acquired. He tries to show how out of these urges there develops in the course

of evolution a hierarchy of linguistic symbolisms to reduce its various forms to those primordial needs (Lévi-Strauss, 1953, p. 536; Kluckhohn, 1953, pp. 507 ff.).

Some patterns of rhythmical reiteration can again be quoted as examples showing how what we refer to as syllables owe their origin partly to the urge to suck the mother's breast (Stein, 1949).

I have not mentioned medicine since, as Sir Francis R. Fraser has recently said (Fraser 1960), biology is the larger field of knowledge which includes the lesser field of medicine. The data provided by oto-laryngology, neurology, psychiatry and other branches of medicine are of great value, but these specialities have not made any major contributions to the understanding of the structure of language, its disorders and their treatment. This is obvious in respect of the interaction of biological and sociological factors in human beings generally, as Lord Adrian pointed out not so long ago (Adrian, 1959). What he says holds good also in the case of the "talking" individual.

(7) *Communication theorists* study the rules of the game of communication played by the partners regardless of their culture, status, etc. (Lévi-Strauss, 1953, p. 538). We certainly find our patients obeying strangely encoded rules of the game.

The unit which communication theory investigates is the community and not the individual. The community shares the ability to perceive, register and transmit signals. An example of a signal is the dance of the bee, by which other bees are induced to fly to the place where nectar can be found; or, when an infant utters "papapa" or "mamama" and the like, it probably means to convey something like "I like you, I want you", "come to me", "pick me up". It may be remarked in passing that some of the features of signals, such as clicks and rhythmical reiterations, are, as I have shown in previous publications, genetically fixed (Stein, 1942, 1949). The importance for us of features that need not be learned should therefore be realized.

In addition to the three abilities just mentioned we find the acquired capacity to utilize the signals as elementary tokens for objects and events. Thereby the signals become signs, and the code containing a consistent system of such signs is language (Ruesch, 1959).

To use our last example, when uttering the words *pater* or *mater*, our "father", "mother", the Romans no longer suspected that their ancestors had converted "papapa" and "mamama" into *pater* and *mater* (Weekley, 1930). These words are signs pointing to particular persons, but people did not necessarily use them to induce others to *bring* father or mother.

The language system also contains a type of word called symbol. If, for instance, we trace the syllable "pa" in *pater* back on the developmental and evolutionary time scales we arrive first at "papapa", then at /πa πa πa/, containing the bilabial click /π/, and ultimately at the primary rhythmical sequence /π π π . . . /. These clicks or sucking noises are signals belonging to the body-language system, and indicate affection on the level of "oral eroticism". This can be hinted at pictorially, as, for instance, in this pictogram or hieroglyph of ancient Egyptian. The words that an Egyptian said or wrote were *arbitrary* aggregates of sounds, pictures or letters of a symbolic nature (Fig. 1 from Gardiner, *Egyptian Grammar*, p. 435).

man with hand to mouth

Det. eat, exx. *wnm* 'eat'; *ḥḳr* 'hungry'; drink, ex. *sw(r)i* 'drink'; speak, exx. *sḏd* 'relate'; *gr* 'be silent'; think, ex. *kȝi* 'devise'; feel, ex. *mri* 'love'.

Figure 1

The combinations of sound signs (or phonograms) with the representation of the object as in Figure 1 (pictogram or determinative) and their meanings show how much depended on the code used in the context.

The word symbol itself tells us what I have been illustrating. It consists of the syllable *sym* "together" and *bolon* "that which has been thrown", and this means something perceptible resulting from a mental activity which grips together such things as have something in common. In the terminology of analytical psychology symbols are tallies (like the two broken pieces of bone or coin used in Grecian times for identification) combining the known or familiar with the unknown or "uncanny" bit. In a wider sense a symbol expresses the union of opposites; for instance, the above hieroglyph serves to indicate love and hate, talking and silence, thinking and feeling, deprivation and gratification. The determinative in the form of the man with his hand to his mouth is the image which best expressed the twofold nature of mental and linguistic activity.

(8) Where, it may be asked, in the large field covered by all these sciences does our discipline find its place? Answers to the question have recently been given in three short papers (*Speech Pathology and Therapy* III/2, 1960, pp. 84 ff.). However, the statements made, including those about communication and dynamics, are not explicit enough, because the specificity of the subject, the methods of approach and of validation are not indicated.

Our science must, of course, follow the principles of current scientific methodology. It may legitimately borrow categories, designations and models employed by the sciences mentioned. If, however, it were merely to usurp them (and it has often done so!) it would not get a place of its own, but would rightly have to be grouped with services ancillary to the above mentioned disciplines. Rather is it developing new methods of approach that are adapted to its subject matter and tasks. It endeavours to find and apply its own criteria of relevance for the analysis and classification of the elements. To do this, and to avoid confusion with other professions such as education, elocution, etc., "speech therapy" must produce a technical language fit to make its unique concepts quotable. This should be complemented by a consistent nomenclature defined as a collection of terms that indicate by their design the relation between the concepts and the diagnostic entities in the system.

To say now what our speciality is supposed to do, it may be helpful to outline the admittedly somewhat arbitrary stratification of the procedures involved.

LEVEL I. For the purpose of description it may profitably adopt the rigorous procedures of linguistics.

LEVEL II. The linguistic patterns should then be looked upon from the point of view of anthropology and sociology, so as to ascertain the difficulties facing the patient when confronted with the sanctioned ways in which mankind and social groups cope with certain needs.

LEVEL III. These difficulties can then be analysed on the one hand into elementary inborn drives, categories provided by biology, on the other hand into dynamic patterns, categories used by psychology. These sciences in conjunction with anthropology also throw light on evolutionary processes responsible for changes of linguistic attitudes emerging from the choice of certain oral signals.

LEVEL IV. The models provided by communication theory would then show how the interrelation between signals, signs and symbols affects the patient when playing the game of communication with his partners, regardless of their nature and status.

I have so far shown how we can, in conformity with what other sciences do, take over concepts from other sciences. We do not follow the models built by the teachers of languages since they are normative rather than operational.

LEVEL V is the one on which our profession stands. On it we go beyond the boundaries of linguistic and bio-psychological analysis of utterances, and by integrating what we have taken arrive at assumptions in terms of aggregates of invariants or factors that are not altered by culture patterns.

Our procedure aims at describing images pointing to the primordial patterns of action or archetypes. Statements made to this end should, if they are truly diagnostic, be operational inasmuch as they should involve activities that the patient, having decoded them, can carry out without having been explicitly told or taught.

Such primeval patterns or archetypes are not in themselves observable. To gain understanding and thereby to acknowledge such theoretical entities is admittedly difficult. Mayo (1954) of the University of Birmingham has shown that physical and mental sciences agree that such entities are "real" and "existing", and it should not be suggested that members of our profession lag behind in this ability of comprehension or are in agreement with another philosopher, one Bishop Berkeley

> "Who remarked metaphysically, darkly,
> That what we don't see
> Cannot possibly be,
> And the rest is altogether unlarkly."[1]

Freud's Id and Ego, Jung's Self and the archetypes are not observable, yet are "real" and "existent". They do a job, the

[1] R. F. Ashley-Montagu, *Weekend Book*, Nonesuch Press.

results of which we can observe (Stein, 1965). These entities entail, like symbols in the strict sense, complementary opposites such as black and white, high and low. In the phraseology of communication theory the patterns would be said to have a dichotomous structure or to be "binary coded" (Jakobson, 1956). Psychologists are aware of the two opposite aspects of such entities when they operate with the idea of the person showing simultaneously both male and female, conscious and unconscious aspects, and experiencing pleasure and pain, love and hate.

The very articulateness of language we can trace back to the conjunction of such pairs of opposites, inasmuch as some consonants and the so-called vowels occurring in an utterance are primarily expressive of the evolutionary trend to unite the act of taking good objects in and expelling bad ones (Stein, 1949). The images that hint at the existence of primordial entities are known as motifs or themes, comparable to those in music, of which the composer may, but need not, be aware when composing.

In phonemic analysis Trubetzkoy (Trubetzkoy, 1936) arrived at and Martinet (Martinet, 1949) elaborated the concept of such a theme named the archephoneme. Jakobson maintains that the receiver of linguistic signs – and signals – is always presented with paired alternatives between which he has to choose (Jakobson, 1956). The elements stand in binary opposition, that is, the two phonemic items represent two polar aspects of the archephoneme. Sapir says that a speech sound has no primary singleness of reference (Sapir, 1949). Going further, I maintain that "what is being said" denotes both sameness and otherness, a characteristic well known to psychologists since Plato's time (Jung, 1948, p. 339). That of which the observable data are aspects is, however, not perceptible. Here we have the link between linguistics and dynamic psychology.

The amalgamation of all these concepts into one idea that guides our therapeutic approach justifies the rejection of a statement made by a former Minister of Health, that we "teach the correct use of the organs of speech in the same way that physiotherapists or occupational therapists teach . . . the correct use of muscles injured or impaired by disease". What we do, or should do, is investigate and analyse "what is being said" about primary existent things and how it is said. Ultimately we arrive at an underlying theoretical entity for which Plato, and later Aristotle, used the term *rhema* (from *ereo* "I say"). We should incorporate into our body of knowledge such concepts as phonemes, morphemes, syntagmemes, archephonemes and others. In addition I wish to introduce the new concepts of the *rhememe* and the *arche-rhememe*. The rhememe is the theme which pervades the rhema, that is the actual form of the utterance. The rhememe roughly corresponds to the structure of signals and signs, the model built under the guidance of the observed relationships between the linguistic elements. The arche-rhememe is the archetypal theoretical entity or the dynamic agent which we contrive or stipulate, the backroom boy doing the job of talking, that is, of conveying and registering true linguistic and psychological symbols in the sense of conjunctions of opposites.

The body of knowledge concerned with these should, therefore, be referred to as the science of Rhememes, instead of the misnomer speech therapy. I propose to revive a now obsolete word and call it *Rhematology*.

The Rhematologist is a scientific inquirer who:

1. Makes an adequate observation, description and analysis of the essential structural patterns of an individual's language by a series of definite, rigid and unambiguous operations.

2. Arranges the data in fields and on levels. This allows the ultimate recognition of theoretical entities or factors, that is rhememes and arche-rhememes, which do particular jobs for the speaker.

3. Formulates statistically the most significant factors and their constellations.

4. Evaluates their relevance in the diagnosis and therapy of the individual case (cf. Dubois, 1960).

5. For the purpose of treatment makes diagnostic models of a given disorder which contain the factors assumed to be responsible for the symptoms observed. Therapy consists in the purposive handling of these dynamic agents, that is, theoretical entities, in an effort to predict the operations of these contrivances. In this way the assumptions are tested and flaws in the theory detected which lead to modifications of the theory. Insofar

as the assumptions are verified the disorder is said to be successfully treated.

This is precisely what is by consensus called a "science".

REFERENCES

Lord Adrian (1959) *British Medical Journal* II, p. 78

Brough, J. (1951) "Theories of General Linguistics in the Sanskrit Grammarians", *Transactions of the Philological Society*

Carroll, J. B. (1959) *The Study of Language*, Harvard University Press

Dubois, R. J. (1960) *Mirage of Health*, London, Allen & Unwin

Fraser, F. R. (1960) "The Challenge to the Medical Profession", *British Medical Journal*, p. 1821

Haas, W. (1954, 55) "On Defining Linguistic Units", *Transactions of the Philological Society*

Haas, W. (1957, 58) "The Identification and Description of Phonetic Elements", *Transactions of the Philological Society*

Harris, Z. S. (1951) *Methods in Structural Linguistics*, University of Chicago Press

Hockett, C. F. (1958) *Modern Linguistics*, New York, Macmillan

Jackson, J. H. (1958) *Selected Writings*, London, Staples Press

Jakobson, R. (1956) *Fundamentals of Language*, p. 44, The Hague, Mouton

Jung, C. G. (1948) *Symbolik des Geistes*, Zurich, Rascher

Kluckhohn, C. (1953) *Universal Categories of Culture in Anthropology Today*, ed. Kroeber, Cambridge University Press

Lévi-Strauss, C. (1953) *Social Structure in Anthropology Today* ed. Kroeber, Cambridge University Press

Lubbock, J. (1889) *The Origin of Civilisation*, London, Longmans, Green

Martinet, A. (1936) "Neutralisation et Archiphoneme", *Travaux du Circle Linguistique de Prague*

Mayo, B. (1954) "The Existence of Theoretical Entities", *Science News*

Ruesch, J. (1959) "General Theory of Communication", *American Handbook of Psychiatry*, New York, Basic Books

Sapir, E. (1949) *Selected Writings*, Cambridge University Press

Stein, L. (1942) The Growth and Present State of Speech Therapy, II, *Medical Press*, p. 141

Stein, L. (1942) *Speech and Voice*, London, Methuen

Stein, L. (1949) *The Infancy of Speech and the Speech of Infancy*, London, Methuen

Stein, L. (1956) "Analytical Psychology, a 'Modern' Science", *Journal of Analytical Psychology*, II

Trubetzkoy, N. S. (1936) "Die Aufhebung der phonologischen Gegensätze", *Travaux du Cercle Linguistique de Prague*

Weekley, E. (1930) *Adjectives and Other Words*, London, Murray

3

W. HAAS, Manchester

Signs and Signals

The subject I am to discuss may be treated in a number of ways. It will be found to present, in fact, almost as many facets as there are contributions to the present symposium. The use of verbal signs and signals is a physical and physiological process as well as a psychological one. It may be compulsive or conventional, automatic or learnt. It is a social phenomenon as well as a matter of individual capacity and choice. Again, signs and signals, when we shift our attention from the *uses* of them and turn to examining their *intrinsic nature*, become a subject of linguistic enquiry.

It seemed to me that something worthwhile for speech therapy – though of course not everything – may be discoverable by a linguistic approach. Some of the important new ideas in linguistic studies, especially in phonetics, seem almost to have arisen from concentrating on what I take to be a central issue for us – namely, the *relation* between the *signs* we make, on the one hand, and the *sounds* which signal them, on the other.

A meeting such as ours – of various interests, and of different lines of study – offers opportunities. But it also presents something of a challenge. For my own part, I cannot help being aware of the fact that those recent developments in linguistic studies are viewed by many with feelings of unease – with suspicion that the new (or new-fangled) ideas are difficult, abstruse, inaccessible, or even worse, that they are of no practical use. Perhaps I can do something to dispel this feeling.

Let me try, then, to begin with a clean sheet, as if nothing were known of those new developments, as if things like phonemes and allophones had never been heard of before. It is only by trying to re-define those familiar technical terms, only by trying to introduce them as if they were new, that I can hope to show their significance, and hope to dispel suspicion of them.

Phonetic value. Signals

The best way, perhaps, of coming upon the most important new ideas in phonetic analysis is to become clearly aware of the fact that there can be no such thing as a *complete* description of what we are trying to describe. Having described an utterance, however accurately, we can always seek to be more accurate; we can take account of more and ever more features of speech, make our transcription ever more "narrow". This inevitable incompleteness of description is nothing to be regretted. A mere chase after ever greater exactitude could only – to speak with Bloomfield – "clutter up" our record, and clutter it up, as Saussure said, with "details which in themselves have no value". This raises a most important question – the crucial question of phonetic analysis: Which details *do* have value?

If we cannot have completeness of description, then clearly we must choose *what* to describe. And having to *choose*, we must make sure that our choice is not arbitrary: that we describe such "details" as are worth describing; also, that we *grade* them in some order of relative importance.

The most significant advances of modern linguistics consist precisely in our having become more clearly aware of principles of selection and of grading. We have gained a clearer notion of *phonological values*. This, on the face of it, should be of importance for those who have to treat defects of disorders of speech. It should make for clearer discrimination between what are major defects and what are minor.

Starting, then, with the flow of speech, with given utterances, and making the attempt to describe them – what shall we select as the most important, the most deserving of description? What is it that in fact determines order of importance among the "elements" of speech? The answer comes readily: it is a matter of their importance for communication. The purpose of the variety of noises we make when speaking a language is to convey a variety of messages. Differences of sound, then, the "details" which we distinguish in the general flow of speech, will have value in proportion to their *power of distinguishing messages*, their power of keeping different meanings distinct.

This simple truth is the foundation of modern phonology. "Foundation-truths" ought to be simple. The first thing to notice, among the many things resting on this foundation, is that, in assessing their values, we have to concentrate upon the *differences* between the sundry noises we produce in speaking a language, rather than on the total noises themselves – the differences, and the use of these differences for distinguishing meanings. This functional approach to phonetic description has given us a principle of selection and a technique of analysis which have transformed the whole subject. We are not concerned any more with mere sounds, mere noises, mere physical or physiological facts. We are dealing with sounds that serve a purpose, i.e. with *signals*.

The selection of signals. Distinctive sounds

Our question then must be: Is there a technique of analysis that will ensure selection of the important signals of speech? There is, and again the basic idea is familiar. We want to pick out such differences of sound as are correlated with differences of meaning. We cannot begin, then, with mere "portions of speech": we begin with utterances which "have meaning" ("signs", as the linguists say). For the sake of clarity, let us take first, as such an utterance, a simple word, for example, Bloomfield's *pin*, and consider such minimal substitutions for some segment as will give us other words – words of different meaning from *pin*. By, say, substitution in the initial position, we obtain nine further words:

1. pin
2. bin
3. tin
4. din
5. kin
6. fin
7. θin (*thin*)
8. sin
9. ʃin (*shin*)
10. win

Incidentally, it is sometimes difficult to settle what to regard as a minimal contrastive segment. Shall we regard the prevocalic onset of *gin*, for example, as simple /ǰ/, or as complex /dʒ/? Or consider aspiration, the *h* following the initial *p* in *pin*. Why do we tend to take this aspiration as part of *p*? Such questions require answers, but I shall pass them over now, for I want to concentrate on the broad outlines of the procedure.

The general technique itself has been given various names. We may call it "analysis by CONTRASTIVE SUBSTITUTION". The eminent Danish scholar L. Hjelmslev called it COMMUTATION (a mutation of sound correlated with a mutation of meaning). It gives us what we may call DISTINCTIVE SOUNDS – ten of them in all, in our example. These distinctive sounds form a class – a "substitution class" or PARADIGM; they constitute the class of distinctive sounds which fill the WORD-FRAME or WORD-FUNCTION (-*in*).[1]

We know that the differences between the sounds in this paradigm are important – that is, important for English, though of course not all of them are necessarily important for other languages. They are not even important for every kind of English. For a Cockney speaker, there is no paradigm containing no. 7, *th* /θ/. The Cockney *f* corresponds to both *th* and *f* of Standard English. German will give no paradigms containing Nos. 7 or 10 in comparable positions. If *th* /θ/ occurs it will be as a queer kind of *s*; i.e. it will not contrast with *s* in any German paradigm, but may replace it without alteration of meaning.

Cannot this make a difference for speech therapy? Suppose a German-speaking child has a lisp; is this at all the same sort of defect as when an English-speaking child has one? Surely, in English children, this is a far more serious defect; they would be confusing two distinctive sounds, and hence different meanings: giving us only one of any pair such as *thing* ÷ *sing*, *thick* ÷ *sick*, *mouth* ÷ *mouse*, *think* ÷ *sink*, etc. A lisp has higher priority for treatment in an English-speaking child than a child speaking, say, German or French. Similar considerations apply to all those cases which speech therapists are used to calling "substitutions". They need to be evaluated. To confuse /s/ and /ʃ/ (*sh*) is serious in English, but would

---

[1] Read: "blank, *in*". Terms which are to be used with a special technical meaning are introduced in capital letters.

be of little importance if you had to speak Japanese. In normal Japanese speech the two sounds do occur, but they never contrast; they do not appear in one and the same paradigm; they are never commutable. This is one example of how the simple technique of "commutation" supplies us with criteria of relevance.

The description of distinctive sounds

We select, then, sounds which serve to distinguish meanings – elements of DIACRITICAL POWER. Having selected them, we proceed to describe them. But how are we to describe such sounds? They have all sorts of characteristics – some more, some less important. We want to describe chiefly what is most important about them, what distinguishes one from any other among the members of a paradigm (substitution-class). Most important about p, in our paradigm, is what distinguishes it from b, t, d, etc. – that is, from all the other nine. Most important about a distinctive sound are its DISTINCTIVE FEATURES, i.e. features, in terms of which we can describe all its contrasts. There are $\frac{n(n-1)}{2}$ contrasts for n members of a paradigm – 45 in our example.

For the purpose of *indicating* the distinctive features, in terms of which we describe the distinctive sounds, we commonly make use of the tools of traditional phonetics. We do so in a selective manner. We fall back upon the framework of the organs of speech in order to choose some scheme of categories – articulatory categories such as "voice", "position of articulation", "degree of obstruction", etc. – in terms of which we can describe the given contrasts. This is more or less like other procedures of contrastive description – say, a fruit grower's method of dealing with apples. Having chosen categories such as colour, size, taste, in terms of which he can describe contrasts between the different kinds of apple, he proceeds to group them as "red large and sweet", "yellow small and spicy", and "green large and sour", etc. In like manner, we proceed to characterize our distinctive sounds under chosen articulatory categories. The method is familiar. Under the category of voice, for instance, the contrast of p with b is interpreted as "voiceless" *versus* "voiced"; under the category of articulatory position, p is contrasted with t as "labial" *versus* "alveolar"; under the category of degree of obstruction, *p* is contrasted with *f*, as "stop" *versus* "fricative". Schematically,

$$p \begin{array}{c} \div b \\ \div t \\ \div f \end{array} = \begin{pmatrix} \text{vl} \\ \text{lab.} \\ \text{stop} \end{pmatrix} \begin{array}{c} \div \text{v} \\ \div \text{alv.} \\ \div \text{fric.} \end{array}^{1}$$

In this way, we have characterized the distinctive sound *p* without being arbitrary about it. It is described by *a bundle of distinctive features*: *p* is voiceless, labial and stop. Do we need any more features or more categories? There are six more contrasts of *p* in our paradigm. Can we account for them without adding to the features of *p*? We find that *p* differs from *k* as "labial" from "velar", that it differs from *d* as "labial and voiceless" from "alveolar and voiced", and so on. We find that we do not need to add to the characteristics of *p*, or to the categories under which its contrasts are interpreted, in order to account for all its differences in the paradigm. The same sound, in another language, may of course have to be characterized by different features. In Russian, for instance, most consonants will require another category of two features; they may be "hard" or "soft" (palatalized), e.g. /brat/ "brother" as distinct from /brat′/ "to take"

What, now, about the occurrences of similar sound-signals in other positions, within the same language? How, for instance, shall we describe the initial in *play* or the medial in *apt*? Are they similar enough to the initial of *pin* to let them pass as sounds of the same type? This cannot be taken for granted. What is "similar enough"? To the ears of a Chinese, these sounds in *play* or *apt* are more like the *b* in *bin* than like the *p* in *pin*. Are we sure that an English child who is acquiring his "native tongue" might not make the identifications of the Chinese? Might he not confine his discrimination between *p* and *b*, so-called, to those positions in which *p* is aspirated, as it is in *pin*? And then, might he not confuse *blot* and *plot*, *blunder* and *plunder*, *blank* and *plank*, etc., though being perfectly able to distinguish *bin* from *pin*? Observation even of moderate accuracy tells us that the sounds which we have learned to regard as instances of *p* are in fact very different. In contrast to the aspiration and

[1] Read: "*p* differs from *b* as *voiceless* from *voiced*," etc.

central plosion of the *pin*-instance, those which occur in *play* or *apt* have no aspiration, the first has "lateral plosion", and the second is not exploded at all. How important are these differences? How important for English? To discover the answer, we apply commutation to the new cases; we ask whether "unaspirated", "lateral plosion" or "unexploded" are required for the description of contrasts in the new paradigms. We consider substitutions for the blank

– l e i		a – t	
p – – –	(play)	– p –	(*apt*)
k – – –	(clay)	– k –	(*act*)
f – – –	(flay)	– f –	(*aft*)
s – – –	(slay)	– n –	(*ant*)

Clearly, we can interpret these contrasts in terms of the same bundle of distinctive features, "voiceless labial stop". Even the new contrast of our *p* with *n* would be interpreted as a contrast of "stop", namely "stop" ÷ "nasal" ("complete obstruction" *versus* "nasal opening"). The significant distinctions can all be made with reference to the same three features – voiceless labial stop. This recurrent bundle of distinctive features, which characterizes a large number of distinctive sounds, is called the PHONEME /p/. The many distinctive sounds which are characterized in this way, and which are otherwise different, are called ALLOPHONES, or allophonic variants, *of the same phoneme*. Each is said to "represent" the same phoneme, also, to "belong" to the same phoneme-class.

There are, again, a number of more special problems about this phonemic characterization of distinctive sounds, and about their grouping: problems concerning sameness or difference of features, and problems concerning sameness or difference of meaning. For example, we may ask about meanings: does the strong aspiration of emphatic speech signal a difference of meaning? Or, about features: what about the *t* of, say, *eighth* /-tθ/ which is not alveolar but dental? Does it represent another phoneme than the *t* of *eight*? My answer to both questions is "No". But I should say that such an answer is not obvious. There are also problems concerning the choice of features most suited for the description. It is better, for instance, to characterize the instances of English /p/ as "stop" than to characterize them as "plosive". Though most of them have both features, "stop", as we have seen, has the wider distribution. Once more, I do not wish to go into such special problems now, but must keep to the broad outlines of the analytic procedure.

Grades of importance

We have seen what it is that is supremely important about the sounds of a language – their diacritical value. This attaches to their distinctive features, to those bundles of them, the phonemes, which are embodied or represented by the various distinctive sounds, each phoneme being identifiable in a whole class of them. It remains to introduce some gradation in importance among the elements which have been selected for description.

Of the differences among phonemes and phonemic features, some are more, some less important. Phonemic contrasts which occur frequently, in comparable contexts of utterance and situation, are more important than contrasts which more rarely do so. For example, r and l or k and t contrast more frequently in English than, say, r and w or $\int$ and $\mathfrak{z}$. How many minimal contrasts $\int \div \mathfrak{z}$ can we find? How likely are these in the same utterance-frame? We say that the contrasts $r \div l$ or $k \div t$ carry a heavier FUNCTIONAL LOAD. This gradation, too, should be significant for determining priorities for treatment.

We have also seen that, in addition to its distinctive and phonemic features, a distinctive sound has many less important features such as the aspiration, implosiveness, lateral plosion, etc., of some allophones of the phoneme /p/. We shall not say that difference of allophones is just unimportant. It is *less* important. Yet there are degrees of importance. Here we must make a further distinction – a distinction of two kinds of allophone, CONDITIONED and OPTIONAL.

(*a*) *Conditioned allophones* (AUTOMATIC VARIANTS). Their differences are conditioned by different environments, i.e. they never occur in the same position. They occur, as some have expressed it, in COMPLEMENTARY DISTRIBUTION, i.e. in mutually exclusive frames. Obvious examples are the English allophones of the phoneme /l/, the clear [l] occurring initially before vowels, the dark [ɫ], in other positions. The distinguishing "conditioned" features are of some importance here, though less important than the phonemic ones. They signal the environment. For example, a clear *l*, as also an aspirated stop, helps to signal boundaries of syllables and often of words. Also, since aspiration occurs only with voiceless consonants in the English language, it supports the perception of the important and distinctive feature, voicelessness, and may even deputize for it.

(b) *Optional allophones* (or FREE VARIANTS). These do occur in the same frames, but they do so *without* correlation of their differences with semantic contrasts; we may replace one by another without altering the meaning. For example, an *r* may be rolled or not rolled or more or less rolled. We do, in fact, all speak differently, each pronouncing different allophones within the range of permissible variation. The "optional" features which distinguish such "free variants" are of course less important than either the phonemic or the conditioned allophonic features.[1]

From this gradation it is clear what should follow in treating defective speech. Failure to discriminate between phonemic features and phonemes is a serious error, especially if their contrasts carry a heavy functional load. Failure to discriminate conditioned features and allophones comes next, and free variants hardly matter; we need only trouble about them if the variation comes near to confusing phonemes, or (as may also happen) when we have some aesthetic objections, say, against a harsh voice, or against speaking through the nose, and the like. A lisp, we have seen, is only aesthetically objectionable in a French or a German child; confusion of *s* and *ʃ* is only a confusion of conditioned allophones in Japanese speech: both are more serious in English. Or take my own pronunciation of English. Having learned English late in life and in a hurry, I am very far indeed from being perfect. I hope to be intelligible, that is, I hope that I have mastered the distinctive features of English, but I know that I am far from having mastered all the conditioned features of the language. And occasionally, an individual free variant of mine comes near to transgressing the SAFETY-MARGIN between two phonemes. For example, my /w/, though bilabial like that of Standard English, tends to be pronounced without lip-rounding and velarity; it can therefore come dangerously near to the labio-dental *v*, without quite being that. The notion of

[1] Free variants, which are not characterized by the same distinctive features, might be referred to as "allophonemes".

the "safety-margin" between different phonemes and between different distinctive features is again a very useful one.

In view of the importance we find in our gradation of phonetic value it is desirable that we should make clear, in a phonetic transcription, what differences we wish to take account of – only phonemic or also allophonic. In a "broad" transcription (marked as a rule by being enclosed between diagonals) we shall be content to distinguish phonemes, e.g. have only one symbol /p/ for the different allophones all of which are characterized as voiceless labial stops. Our traditional transcriptions are not quite consistent in this respect. They keep to a principle of phonemic distinction, when dealing with stop sounds; i.e. they refrain here from assigning different symbols to the different allophones. But they persist in assigning different symbols to clear /l/ and dark /ł/, which never contrast with one another and are characterized by the same distinctive features. This inconsistency is confusing and can have undesirable practical consequences. For example, I am told that there are teachers of English in the Far East who will expend much energy in trying to teach a Japanese the difference between clear and dark /l/, when he has not yet mastered the difference between /l/ and /r/, these being allophones of the same phoneme in Japanese. To teach in this way is to ignore priorities. I should not be surprised if such errors crept in occasionally among conscientious language-teachers as well as speech therapists. Our transcriptions seem to ask for it; they present the difference of /l/-allophones as something quite as important as that between /l/ and /r/, or between any other phonemes. If we were to teach Polish or to treat a Polish child, the difference between clear /l/ and dark /ł/ would be highly important for the two do contrast in Polish; they are commutable: for example, *lava* in Polish means "lava", while *tava* means "a bench", *laska* – "a rod", and *taska* – "grace". What is highly important in one language need not be equally important in another, and other transcriptions should take account of this fact.

Types of defect

The problems of teaching a foreign language seem to be sometimes similar, in some ways, to the problems of remedial training in the native tongue. I stress "sometimes" and "in some ways"; we must not overlook the differences. But such analogies as there are seem to be instructive.

The patient may have to learn much the same things as the pupil. With both of them it is important to see that deviation from what is wanted is rarely capricious. In order to see this, we require an exact diagnosis of the defects; and the subtler organization that has been brought into phonetic analysis permits such diagnosis. It enables us to discover some clear-cut types and regularities of deviation. We are dealing here with the description of the deviations themselves, not with their causes – with *what* is wrong, rather than *why* it is wrong. The discovery and removal of causes does of course require help from other disciplines – from physiology, neurology, psychology.

First, there may be difficulty in producing a certain *distinctive* feature. For example, a child may have no velarity for any of its consonants, just as, say, a Frenchman learning English would find that "interdental" as in English *th*, is absent from his native inventory of distinctive features. Or it may be that the features are present, but a particular *combination* of them in a phoneme causes difficulty. For example, the combination of "nasal" and "velar" /ŋ/ as in the medial consonant of *singer*, may be found difficult, while "nasal" would combine easily with "labial", /m/, and "velar" with "stop", /k/ – just as for an Englishman learning German or Welsh it would be difficult to effect the simultaneous pronunciation of "velar" and "fricative" in, say, the final of *bach*, although he would of course be familiar with both these features in other combinations.

Even more frequently, patient and pupil are perfectly able to pronounce the distinctive features and distinctive sounds correctly, but unable to discriminate between them in the required way. They may treat them as allophonic variants, that is, they may treat them either as conditioned variants – in the way in which a Spaniard, for instance, would tend to treat English /d/ and /ð/, which he can pronounce, but normally in different frames (in complementary distribution) – or they may treat them as free variants, that is, as if the option between them were free. Exact diagnosis, here, should help us to choose the most effective remedial exercises – exercises of the sounds in the *critical frames*.

Finally, different phonemes, though correctly pronounced and recognized as different, may have their contrast and discrimination inappropriately limited to certain positions and therefore reduced in importance. A native English speaker finds it difficult to distinguish /k/ from /t/ or /g/ from /d/ in initial position before /l/: /tliːn dlʌvz/ sounds to him like /kliːn glʌvz/. He cannot easily hear the difference between, say, Czech *tlapky* "little paws" and *klapky* "blinkers". A German or a Russian, again, learning English will have no difficulty in pronouncing and properly distinguishing voiced from voiceless consonants in initial and medial positions; but in final position he will tend to pronounce voiceless consonants only: he will tend to put *rip* for both "rip" and "rib", *lice* for both "lice" and "lies", *rot* for both "rot" and "rod", *wick* for "wick" and "wig". We say that, for him, the phonemic contrast is NEUTRALIZED in some positions. Its functional load is reduced to what it is in German or Russian. In teaching, we should locate, and then concentrate on these positions. Are there not parallel cases in speech therapy? This touches upon another field of phonetic study, which I can only refer to briefly: namely, what we may call PHONOTACTIC and PROSODIC studies.

Phonotactic and prosodic features

Every language comprises certain habits or rules, not only for the formation of its distinctive sounds, but also for their *combination*: phonotactic rules. These rules are analagous to those operative on the phonetic level and to the syntactic ones at work on the grammatical level.

To illustrate briefly: If I ask "Do you know what *strimps* are?" you will say "No", but think it possible that I have used an unfamiliar English word. If, on the other hand, I ask what a /ʃtrumpf/ is, you know immediately that this cannot possibly be an English word, though the single sounds are familiar. (It is, in fact, German for "stocking".) Now, speech-defects may consist, as we all know, in failure to master the phonotactics of the language, rather than failure to pronounce its individual sounds. For example, they may concern only certain clusters of consonants – the kind of failure which is familiar to an Englishman learning German or Russian. Here, too, precise analysis should help us clearly to diagnose what sort of defect we are dealing with, and what sort of exercise is called for.

Lastly, there are prosodic features extending over larger units – stress-patterns, pitch-contours, and the like – which may also cause difficulty. These (as well as some other features) are often of great importance even though they may have very little contrastive use, or none at all. Their importance may lie in that they *organize* the given sentences, phrases, words – rather than distinguish them from others: they may determine boundaries between the distinctive units, or mark them as belonging to important grammatical categories and constructions. If they have themselves no contrastive use, they may serve to *determine typical frames* for other elements to contrast in. By catching the mere tone-contour or stress-pattern of a word or phrase, I may have half understood it. The choice among possible distinctive sounds for filling the pattern is already very limited. More work needs to be done on these aspects of speech – on elements of DETERMINANT POWER. We all know how seriously communication may be impaired by faulty tone or inappropriate emphasis.

If we tried to sum up, in a few words, the changes that have come into phonetic studies during the last thirty years, we might say this:

Modern phonetics has gone beyond the old task of presenting mere inventories of sounds. We are not content with sound-material, parcelled out in articulatory rubrics. Modern functional phonetics describes an *instrument* – a highly-organized signalling instrument. This instrument consists substantially in regular patterns of human behaviour. Its power and use is that of a social institution – some parts of it being more vital to its functioning than others, but all being kept in balance, all interacting in a subtle gradation of performances.

It must be of some significance for those who treat defects in the use of this subtle instrument that they are able now with greater precision to spot where the faults lie, and able, therefore, to direct their treatment at the critical points. The main contribution of modern linguistics to speech therapy is, I think, a contribution to more exact diagnosis, and to a proper assessment of priorities in the treatment of defects and disorders.

4

J. L. M. TRIM, Cambridge

....

Linguistics and Speech Pathology

Linguistics may claim to be one of the oldest of the social sciences. Early in the nineteenth century Jakob Grimm said that he would prefer a single fact to a thousand refined speculations and since 1870 linguists have been developing and refining their techniques for the observation and recording of spoken utterances and for the analysis and description of the complex linguistic organization which underlies them. In doing so, descriptive linguistics has based itself upon the description of utterances produced by speakers who function normally in their speech community. It is taken for granted that speech is a stable, regularly repetitive activity. Given this, speech is found to provide a complex pattern of closely interrelated utterances. These patterns of interrelation are statable as "the system" of a particular language, and the descriptive linguist predicts that utterances produced by speakers of the language will conform to this system. If his predictions are proved false, he does not require the speakers to reform, but rather amends his grammar! Anyway, the essence of what is termed the structural approach to descriptive linguistics is to focus attention on patterning, on the systems of units of different ranks, operating at different linguistic levels, rather than looking at language as an indefinite agglomeration of individual facts.

The kinds of question we ask on the phonological level for instance are: what are the phonemes of this language? In what environments do they occur? By what allophones are they represented in these environments? How are they related phonetically? i.e. what auditory discriminations are required for the recognition of one rather than another, and what articulatory differences are necessary to produce these? What syllables are there? and what syllable types, involving what classes of phoneme, in what positions and combinations? We can then trace the combination of syllables into feet, into rhythm groups, into intonation groups of increasing complexity, each unit organizing units of lower rank into a characteristic structure.

It is not in phonology alone, however, that such concepts and procedures (developed in detail by W. Haas in Chapter 3) are helpful. The questions to be asked in the course of grammatical analysis are almost literally parallel: i.e. What are the *morphemes* of this language? In what environments do they occur? By what *allomorphs* are they there represented? What *words* and word types are there, involving what classes of morpheme, in what positions and combinations? We can then trace the combinations of words into phrases, clauses and sentences of increasing complexity, each unit organizing classes of units of lower rank into a characteristic structure. By the time all these questions are answered, a pretty good picture of the structure of a language has been built up. In addition, there is of course the lexical question of which sequence of phonemes, or morphemes, goes to make up a particular word. All told, this represents a fairly complex organization. Building up and maintaining an organization of this complexity, and using it to produce and receive individual messages, near-infinite in number, is probably the most complicated task human beings tackle. As we are very well aware, of course, there are so many neuro-muscular systems involved, requiring very exact coordination and synchronization, that there is plenty to go wrong along the line in the series of events (each triggered off by its fore-runner) which constitute the Speech Event.

We may perhaps at this point look at the general outline of the Speech Event.

The speech event proper may be said to start when some stimulus prompts a speaker to initiate a message. In the light of his previous experience and of the present situation he draws upon his store of linguistic knowledge to formulate a linguistic text. He may select a ready-made formula to meet a set, recurrent situation, or pick his way through a maze of choices to match a complex thought with a complex utterance. As the test is formulated, the patterns of motor nerve impulses are organized to bring into play the complex musculature which moves the speech organs to produce sound-waves. This process is largely regulated by the speaker's awareness, through his sensory nerves, of the movements he makes and the sounds they produce. The existence of "sub-vocal speech" which need not involve any muscular movement may indicate an earlier "feed-back", but little, if anything, is known of this. The speech waves impinge upon the listener, producing mechanical vibrations in the air-spaces, bones and fluids of his ears. These stimulate the auditory nerve and the nerve impulses arriving at the brain give rise to the primary perception of sound quality, strongly influenced by contextual factors. The listener uses these perceptions, in conjunction with his linguistic knowledge and observation of the context, to identify the linguistic text concerned. At this point the speech event proper may be said to be concluded, and its success measured by the identity of the text formulated with that identified. The speaker has still, of course, to interpret the text in the light of his previous experience of partly or wholly similar texts, his knowledge and observation of the speaker and other relevant factors in the situation, and to decide what response, if any, is required.

In outline, this process is sufficiently well-known, but it seems to me that to build up a detailed picture of the process, to refine it, to ensure that the processes shown are real and to find out just how they take place, is an important part of human knowledge. As a pupil of Professor Fry, I would indeed regard it as an important, if not the principal aim of the linguistic sciences. In building up this picture, linguistics and phonetics on one side, and logopaedics on the other, have a great deal to contribute and to learn. A malfunction can be evaluated only when set against normal function, but on the other hand, the way the normal human being functions in the speech event is not at all easy to establish. We tend to take all well-run services rather for granted, whether it be a railway system, a television set or the appearance of laundered shirts in one's drawer. Language processes too, if efficient, are liable to be overlooked, being in any case difficult or impossible to observe directly.

This applies above all to the very complicated events in the central nervous systems of speaker and hearer which precede and follow audible speech. The most important sources of information are the results of linguistic analysis of a corpus of utterances and the clinical observations of speech pathologists and of brain surgeons. The latter, in spite of the unique opportunities afforded, have as yet been less rewarding than might have been hoped. As E. H. Lenneburg of Harvard University and the Children's Medical Centre, Boston, observed in his review of Penfield and Roberts "Speech and Brain Mechanisms" (*Language* 36, 1, p. 112). "[Other topics] are only mentioned incidentally. In the latter category is, for instance, the actual nature of the speech disturbances. This is precisely the area that would particularly interest linguists, and where their skills in language analysis might produce important clinical and theoretical discoveries. But the book makes only a few superficial statements about the phonological derangements of aphasic or electrically stimulated patients and there is no mention whatever that morphology or syntax were or were not affected in the utterances of their patients".

The principal features of a linguistic approach to speech disorders would seem to me to be first, exact observation and recording of the patient's speech; secondly, the analysis of the linguistic system which is being operated by the patient, in cases of developmental disorder, or determination of the linguistic levels affected, and to what extent, in cases of traumatic or degenerative disorder. Thirdly, as exact as possible a localization of the malfunction in the patient and the tracing of its ramifications throughout the speech events in which he participates; the assessment, in fact, of its linguistic effect.

The first of these principles is fundamental to all effective work in speech. For this purpose a sound phonetic training is indispensable. Fortunately this fact is well recognized by the College of Speech Therapists. The standard required of and attained by most student therapists is high, and will, I trust, remain so. Constant practice is necessary, of course, but if the practising therapist knows the method, the material and opportunity are always to hand! To illustrate the value of the second and third points to the therapist and also the value of the pathologist's findings for the development of linguistic theory, we may perhaps apply them to a number of speech disorders.

They may certainly be fruitfully employed over the entire field of dyslalia. To insist that a diagnosis of dyslalia be kept entirely free from social and aesthetic judgements upon the speaker's dialect is now unnecessary, in this country, though a reading of the sections on dyslalia in Arnold and Luchsinger's *Lehrbuch der Stimm-und Sprachheilkunde* shows that this is not everywhere the case. I have suggested elsewhere (*Speech*, 1953) ways in which the International Phonetic Association's alphabet may be used in the notation of defective speech. Structural concepts seem, however, scarcely yet to have been applied in this field. If one takes the memorandum on terminology produced by the College of Speech Therapists in 1959, one finds dyslalia defined as: "Defects of articulation or slow development of articulatory patterns including substitutions, distortions, omissions and transpositions of the sounds of speech." Literal paraphrasia (surely phonetic or phonemic would be better!) is defined as "inaccurate use of sounds; changes in the sound patterns of words". I think you will agree that this sounds very much a matter of the fate of individual sounds in individual words, taking the standard language of the community as a point of reference. The causes of dyslalia are then listed as "deficient intelligence, emotional disturbance or immaturity, and the imitation of abnormal patterns of articulation". Dyslalia is shown as a disorder of articulation, as opposed to a disorder of language or speech. Is the speech produced by the dyslalic in fact erratic and devoid of system, best treated by the patient teaching of individual sounds and the correct pronunciation of individual words?

Surely in many cases of infantile dyslalia the child has constructed for himself a well-balanced phonological system which is related to that of the adult world about him, but less complex. A reduced system of this kind will be reasonably adequate to the limited situations of a child's home life. Contextual information, being concrete and accessible, contributes more than its fair share to successful recognition, while adults and older children are adept at learning and speaking the new language. Most children presumably graduate from a rudimentary to a fully developed phonological system, though normal development is so rapid that the stages are fleeting and difficult to assess. Moreover, whereas the adult has relatively stable speech habits and an equally developed system as speaker and as listener, with the young child auditory discrimination must of necessity be more developed than his articulatory skills, since the latter presuppose the former. Neither alone can be taken to represent the child's language. Each must be separately assessed. We need to know, in assessing a child's speech development, to what differences he can respond, as well as those he can reproduce. Auditory under-discrimination (not necessarily a result of hearing deficiency) seems here the more important, since it sets a limit to the child's active speech development. Given full auditory discrimination, normal speech production may be a matter of skill in coordination which time and proper motivation will achieve. It may be that some dyslalias result from a premature stabilization of the phonological system, perhaps because of its very coherence. The longer it continues, the more fixed the speech habits become, and the child may, like most adults, learn to equate what he hears with what he says, and become insensitive to differences he does not employ. There would be considerable fundamental linguistic importance in a series of detailed phonological analyses of normal and dyslalic children, to find out whether development unfolds in a relatively fixed order, whether a coherent system emerges at each stage, and whether dyslalias fall into definable types. In this respect the work of Joy and Robert Albright (1957) and of the English group whose work is reported in Chapters 15, 16 and 17 is of great pioneering value.

With traumatic and degenerative disorders affecting peripheral organs, there will probably be little profit from erecting a special phonological system for the patient. He continues to formulate and identify linguistic texts as before, but experiences difficulty in establishing successful speech events with other people. We may, however, gain clarity by assessing these difficulties in linguistic terms.

Disorders of nasality provide an example: as a distinctive feature, nasality is confined, in English, to the consonant system, in which it distinguishes between b d g and m n ŋ. In cases of hyper- or hypo-rhinophonia, this distinction will be diminished, and listeners will be likely to make false identifications, recognizing nasals or plosives on the basis of clues they are used to. Careful listening and the use of context will restore the position in moderate cases. In severe cases, the distinction may be lost, in which case the linguistic system is reduced, under-differentiated, and intelligibility will depend on context. False identifications will be corrected if this is necessary to ensure that the whole utterance makes sense in its context. If more than one identification is possible in the full context, error is likely.

The effects of hypernasality are more extensive, since the fricative/plosive distinction presupposes a nasal closure. Both tend to be replaced by voiceless nasal fricatives, though a little more differentiation is attainable by the use of a glottal stop or fricative, or both.

The vowel system in English is unaffected, as opposed, say, to that of French or particularly of Portuguese. One would predict that in these languages the intelligibility of speech would be more adversely affected by a given degree of palatal malfunction.

Mature adults who retain full control of the central language organization can often overcome the difficulties interposd by traumatic and degenerative disorders involving peripheral organs of speech and hearing by appropriate compensations, as we see in cases of laryngectomy and even glossectomy. Congenital organic deformations may, of course, inhibit the proper development of organized linguistic knowledge, producing something akin to developmental aphasia.

It is undoubtedly the study of aphasia which is the most exciting and challenging for the linguist, since he hopes that by observing in detail the speech of the aphasic he may be able to deduce something of the way in which utterance is organized in the brain. For instance, is the "Store of linguistic knowledge" physically represented in the brain? Is this store damaged or is access to and from it affected, or are aphasias corresponding to all three conditions found? Do different kinds of aphasia indicate some physical basis for the different levels of linguistic analysis: phonology, lexicon and grammar? Enough is implied by published case-histories and proposed classifications to show that there is indeed some basis, but because the reports and classifications have not been linguistically oriented, the evidence is fragmentary and does not give any picture of the effect on fine structure. Is there evidence, say, for any hierarchical ordering of levels, or for the hierarchical ranking of units at the same level? The terms "nominal aphasia" and "agrammatism" are widely used, but they are vague portmanteau terms and difficult to interpret. Is "nominal aphasia" used for any kind of lexical disorder? Do such disorders affect words at random through the vocabulary?

Or are particular parts of speech affected? Are the "open" word-classes (noun, verb, adjective, adverb) differently affected from the "closed" (prepositions, interrogatives, auxiliaries, articles, etc.)? Within the class of, say, nouns, are words affected randomly, or in "fields" dealing with certain areas of experience? Are word-finding difficulties related to frequency of occurrence? As to agrammatism, what kinds of taxeme (grammatical device) are affected? The ordering of elements? All elements, or any in particular? Of morphemes within words, or only of words within phrases? Or of phrases within clauses? Are grammatical inflections omitted or confused? Any of them more so than others? In cases of jargon, what structure is to be found, and how does it relate to the patient's previous language?

In fact, the topic of aphasia abounds with questions, the answers to which would provide fundamental insights into the workings of human language. In many cases, of course, damage is too extensive to have any differentiating value. The behaviour of the patient is often too unstable for observations carried out over any period of time to be regarded as describing the same condition. Nevertheless, this study clearly affords a virtually unexplored territory of indefinite extent and complexity, inspiring, as such territories do, an intense feeling of excitement and hopelessness mixed in almost equal proportions.

Stammering is widely considered to be a symptom of a deepset emotional disorder, the exact nature of the symptom being of secondary importance. There is a growing body of evidence, however, that whatever the ultimate psychological causes may be, the immediate disorder is of the "feed-back", monitoring control. The improvement brought about by delayed side-tone has been shown (Marland 1957, Nessel 1958) to be of a different order to that produced by masking or other diversionary effects. It is, of course, probable that "stammering" comprises a number of different disorders. If so, differential diagnosis may be helped by a more exact description of the stammerer's speech, noting the particular points in structure at which breakdowns occur, and the units with which they are associated, whether phonetic (e.g. all plosives, or all nasals), phonological (e.g. consonants in initial position in stressed or nuclear syllables) or grammatical (open word-classes occurring at points of choice). One would then be able to establish whether a particular pattern of disturbance was constant for one speaker. If so, it might prove possible to group stammerers into types on this basis and perhaps establish correlations with other characteristics.

I would not wish it to appear that I viewed the linguistic approach I have outlined as a panacea, or even of universal usefulness. It should certainly never exclude other viewpoints. The developed linguistic code we term "English" is superimposed in our speech upon many more primitive – perhaps more vital and fundamental – levels of expression. To a distinguished foreign lecturer who informed the College that it was pointless to teach an Englishman clicks, since they did not occur in English, I once felt constrained to reply with a reduplicated alveolar click /ʇʇ/, our usual form of gentle reproof! The complex interplay of the linguistic and extra-linguistic in speech is clearly exemplified in voice therapy. Whether a speaker uses breathy voice, creaky voice or clear voice throughout his speech is irrelevant in English. "The sun is shining" will be identified as precisely the same text, said with any of these voice qualities. This does not mean that voice quality is unimportant to an Englishman. "Oh darling, I love you!" may depend for its effectiveness on breathy rather than creaky voice; the use of one quality rather than another may be part of a psycho-somatic syndrome, or held to be one by other people; a bright quality may be a more efficient carrier of acoustic information than a breathy or muffled quality and therefore of more use to a public speaker (though not for a tête-à-tête in a quiet restaurant); aesthetic considerations may prescribe one and proscribe another in singing or the speaking of verse; a pathologist may recognize a particular voice quality as a sign of a pathological condition, or conducive to one; one type of voice production, producing one particular quality, may be more economical of effort – as can be seen very clearly from the comparison in the Bell film of the vocal cords in action of a trained with an untrained voice. For all these reasons, and doubtless more besides, voice training and voice therapy are important in England and yet distinctions of voice quality are irrelevant to English. In some languages of South-East Asia, on the other hand, voice quality is an inherent feature of words, serving to distinguish one from another. In the Burmese word -leː'mĩː, for instance, falling tone, nasalized vowel and breathy voice are all inherent distinctive features, present whenever the word is pronounced. Clearly, a Burmese therapist would have to work along different lines. Questions of the comparative efficiency, economy, beauty, social acceptability, of the differing voice qualities do not arise. Instead, they are meaningful, distinctive sound-features which must all be acquired and kept as distinct as possible.

I hope it has been possible to demonstrate that linguistics and speech pathology and therapy have a good deal to contribute to each other. In a way, it is surprising that a meeting has been so long postponed. On the other hand, despite the late Professor J. R. Firth's insistence that what order we find in language is maintained only by human beings in action, and Bloomfield's profession of behaviourism, linguists, jealous of their autonomy, have been very incurious as to how their work contributes to our knowledge of what happens when people talk. The medical profession, on the other hand, bound by its division of responsibility between psychologist, psychiatrist, brain surgeon and oto-rhino-laryngologist, has seemed to an outsider to take a rather simple view of language and speech as a fairly straightforward business of symbolizing ideas by organized patterns of articulation, and has had little use for structural concepts or for a whole view of the speech event.

Now, however, there are many signs, in many countries that speech pathology (or morbid linguistics) affords a meeting ground, and at some time the profession may wish to consider how best to encourage this development. Professor Grewel, when he spoke to us a few years ago, was of the opinion that language disorders should be tackled by teams including medical specialists, therapists and a linguist. In major research clinics this is an excellent proposal; it is possible, clearly, only on a restricted scale. Yet the concepts involved are so simple, and of such general application, that the College might think it worth-while to have all therapists provided with some linguistic equipment.

REFERENCES

Jakobson, R. and Halle, M. (1956) *Fundamentals of Language*, Pt. II
Lenneberg, E. H. (1960) Review of Penfield and Roberts: "Speech and Brain Mechanisms", *Language* **36**, 1

Kandler, G. (1960) "Linguistische Deutung zentraler Sprachstörungen" in *Current Problems in Phoniatrics and Logopaedics* **1**

Borel-Maisonny, S. "Rôle des Concepts phonologique et phonétique dans la structuration de la parole", ibid.

Grewel, F. (1957) "Possession of Language, Use of Language and Speaking", *Speech 2* **21**, 1

Greene, M. (1960) "Diagnosis and Treatment of Late Speech and Language Development in Children", *Folia Phoniatrica* **12**, 2

Kainz, F. (1954–60) *Psychologie der Sprache* **I–IV**

Fry, D. B. (1960) "Linguistic Theory and Experimental Research", *Trans. of the Philological Soc.*

Butfield, E. (1958) "Rehabilitation of the Dysphasic Patient", *Speech Pathology and Therapy* **1**, 1–2

Terminology for Speech Pathology, College of Speech Therapists (1959)

Marland, P. (1957) "Shadowing" – A Contribution to the Treatment of Stammering, *Folia Phoniatrica* **9**, 4

Nessel, E. (1958) "Die Verzögerte Sprachrückkoppelung [Lee-Effekt] bei Stotterern", *Folia Phoniatrica* **10**, 4

Luchsinger, R., and Arnold, G. E. (1959) *Lehrbuch der Stimm-und Sprachheilkunde*, Vienna, Springer

Morley, M. E. (1957) *The Development and Disorders of Speech in Childhood*, Edinburgh, Livingstone

Albright, Joy S. and Robert W. (1957) "The sound-system of an eight-year-old boy", *Maître Phonétique*, No. 107

5

ALAN S. C. ROSS, Birmingham[1]

Historical Linguistics

Linguistics, that is, the Science of Language, which is also often called *Philology*, has two branches: *Descriptive* (or *Synchronic*) Linguistics and *Historical* (or *Diachronic* or *Comparative*) Linguistics. This paper is a brief exposition of Historical Linguistics, which subject may be defined as All consequences arising from two basic statements or axioms.

The first of these axioms is rather easy. It simply states that two languages are *related* if, and only if, they were both once one language. Thus French and Spanish are related because, and only because, they were both once Latin.

This last statement can be put in a variety of ways. We may say "In Spain, that which was Latin has become (*or* has changed into) Spanish"; or, again, "Spanish is descended from Latin", etc. Or, that "Latin is the parent of both Spanish and French", that "Spanish and French are sister-languages", etc. More than two languages can be related; thus, as well as French and Spanish, a number of other languages descend from Latin (e.g. Portuguese, Roumanian, Italian, Provençal, etc.); these are said to form the Romance "family" of languages.

In the case of French, Spanish and Latin, all three members of the family (father and two daughters) are present, but, in the case of most families of related languages, we are not so fortunate. Thus English and German (as well as Dutch, Swedish, Danish, Norwegian, Icelandic, etc.) are related, and form the "Germanic" family; but their parent-language no longer exists, though philologists are able to reconstruct it. In such circumstances it is usual to call the parent-

[1] I am very grateful to Dr L. Stein for his kind help with the preparation of this paper for press.

language by the name of the family with the word *Primitive* prefixed (in this case, then, *Primitive Germanic*).

The first axiom has an implication, namely, that Language Changes. The changes it undergoes follow certain rules, a fact which most people do not realize. Everyone knows, of course, that it is more difficult for an Englishman to read Shakespeare than contemporary English, because of the difference in vocabulary. And most people think that linguistic change is confined to vocabulary.

Changes in vocabulary are, of course, important. They are often due to "borrowing"; thus, for instance, our word *dinner* has been borrowed from French; or – to take a more sophisticated example – when we say *that goes without saying*, we are simply translating French *cela va sans dire*. But there are other kinds of linguistic change more important than change in the vocabulary. These may be classified as (1) Sound-change, (2) Semantic Change, (3) Analogy.

Sound-change

Perhaps the most important type is that illustrated by the following example. In Anglo-Saxon (the language from which Modern English is descended) there are the words *stān*, *bāt* and *rād*. These have changed into Modern English *stone*, *boat* and *road*, respectively – and there are very many other words in which we have an Anglo-Saxon *ā* as against a Modern English [ou]. On the basis of these words we are able to say that there is a sound-change of Anglo-Saxon long *ā* into Modern English [ou]. We can also say, Modern English [ou] derives from Anglo-Saxon long *ā*. (It is usual to write "changes into" as >, "is derived from" as <; thus "AS *ā* > MnE [ou]" or "MnE [ou] < AS *ā*".)

This sound-change (or *sound-law*, to use the term of the nineteenth-century German philologists) has an important implication: every Anglo-Saxon *ā* must give a Modern English [ou] unless special circumstances prevent it doing so. Thus Anglo-Saxon *hālig* follows the law and correctly becomes Modern English ['houli] *holy*, but Anglo-Saxon *hālig dæg* has not become *holy day*, it has become *holiday*. (The explanation is that the vowel was shortened in the Middle English period.)

Some other sound-changes are of a more obvious character. For instance, the Anglo-Saxon language as spoken before A.D. 400 had *l* in its sound-table. We can think of *l* as a consonant in which the tip of the tongue articulates against any point along the median line of the palate. For some reason the articulation of *l* was shifted backwards about 400, so that it adopted a "dark" acoustic character (as it has in the Russian word *loshad* "horse"). It is not easy to pronounce a front vowel before that sound. There were two articulatory attitudes that the Anglo-Saxons could have adopted to overcome the difficulty. They could have shifted the articulation of the front vowel back, thus changing it into a back vowel. Or they could have inserted a back vowel between the back consonant and the front vowel. In fact, both attitudes were implemented. Primitive English **æld* gave, on the one hand, Mercian *ald* (it is from this form that Modern English *old* descends), and, on the other, **æold*, which later gave **æald* (written *eald*) in West Saxon (the language of King Alfred).

Similar influencing of a sound by a neighbouring one is seen in what is called *umlaut*, which is due to the anticipation of the articulation of a vowel during the production of the preceding one. Thus: Welsh plural *meibion* "sons" from an earlier *mab-ion* (*mab* "son"); English *Boulogne* pronounced [bul'ɔin], French [bul'onj]; Primitive Germanic plural **mūsiz* > **mūisi* > Anglo-Saxon *mȳs* (> Modern English *mice*). *Intrusion* of consonant or vowel sometimes occurs when two sounds are in juxtaposition: Anglo-Saxon *þunor*, genitive singular *þunres* > Middle English *þundres*, whence Modern English *thunder*; Primitive English **fugl* > **fugul* > Anglo-Saxon *fugol* (> Modern English *fowl*). *Assimilation* and *dissimilation* are processes by which two neighbouring sounds become more or less like or unlike respectively: Modern English ['dountju] *don't you* > Slang ['dountʃə]; English *pilgrim*, ultimately from Latin *peregrinus*.

Two more kinds of sound-change may be mentioned here. *Loss*, as in Anglo-Saxon *beran* > Middle English *bere* (loss of final *-n*) > Modern English *bear* (loss of final *-e*). In *Metathesis*, two consonants are transposed: Anglo-Saxon *wæps* > Modern English *wasp*, but many dialects have [wɔps], with another metathesis.

The examples given above suggest a two-fold classification of sound-change: isolative (e.g. Anglo-Saxon *stān* > Modern English *stone*, etc.) and combinative (e.g. umlaut). Why do sound-changes happen? The explanation of combinative sound-change is rather obvious, it is simply brought about by the interaction of neighbouring sounds. The many attempts to explain isolative sound-change by correlating it with differences in the structure of the speech-organs, climatic conditions, interaction of two languages, etc., have failed. The only answer that we can give at present is that it is due to *chance*, in the mathematical sense of the word. When a coin is tossed, we say that it is evens whether it falls heads or tails, meaning thereby only that no reason is known to us why it should fall heads rather than tails. But, were we possessed of a full knowledge of the mechanics of the throwing, we should of course *know* whether the coin would fall heads or tails. It is from such considerations that there develops the regarding of chance as "a multitude of unknown causes". Children who are in the process of acquiring their mother-tongue do not copy their parents' or teachers' speech exactly. Thus, when learning the sound [aː], some will err in the direction of [æː], others in the direction of [ɔː]. Provided about the same number err in each direction, the "average" will still be [aː] and there will be no tendency to a sound-change. But if, by chance, there are more who err in the direction of [ɔː] than there are who err in the direction of [æː], there will be a tendency for the sound-change [aː] > [ɔː] to set in.

Semantic change

This concerns the meaning, rather than the structure, of linguistic expressions. Thus the Anglo-Saxon word for "dog" was *hund*. Two developments are to be seen here. First, it is obvious that, in terms of sound, the Modern English word for the animal is not a descendant of its Anglo-Saxon name (the origin of *dog* is, in fact, obscure). Secondly, Anglo-Saxon *hund* has correctly changed into Modern English *hound*, but the meaning of the latter has been restricted to certain kinds of hunting dogs.

Analogy

This is best illustrated by means of grammatical examples. Since Modern English has practically no "grammar", I shall resort to another member of the Germanic family for my first example. In Gothic, the dative plural of *dags* "day" is *dagam*; the dative plural of *nahts* "night" should, correctly, be *nahtim. The actual form is, however, *nahtam*, just like *dagam*, because "night" has been associated with "day", as is very natural. Analogy is a powerful influence in language. Sometimes, it can produce new words, as when Lewis Caroll made up *chortle* by "mixing together" *snort and chuckle*. It can also bring about alterations in the sound- and grammatical systems of a language. Thus, we have the rule that in Modern English *wa* is pronounced [wɔ] (as in *was*), except before gutturals (as in *wag*); the past tense *swam* is thus "irregular" (it should be [swom]) and this is due to analogy with *sit*: past *sat*, where [æ] is regular. Or, to take a grammatical example, the *s*-plural (*dogs*) and the *s*-genitive (*dog's*) of Modern English derive from the Anglo-Saxon endings *-as* and *-es*, respectively; in Anglo-Saxon, these endings were confined to certan classes of nouns (*stān, stānas, stānes* "stone", but *nama, naman, naman* "name"). From these classes these endings "spread" to *all* classes.

After this discussion of linguistic change, we are now in a position to state the Second Axiom of Historical Linguistics, which was referred to on p. 44. This says "Two words of two related languages are said to be *congruent* if and only if they were both once one word in the language which the two related languages both once were". Thus French *pied* and Italian *piede* "foot" are congruent because, and only because, they were both once Latin accusative singular *pedem*. Or, again, English *stone* and Germanic *stein* are congruent because they were both once Primitive Germanic **staina-* (this last is, of course, a reconstructed form, since nothing is preserved of Primitive Germanic).

The fact that Historical Linguistics is defined as All consequences arising from the two axioms, has an important corollary, namely, that anything that cannot be derived from them must, linguistically, be nonsense. Many popular beliefs about language may at once be eliminated by means of this corollary. Thus people often think that related languages must be similar. Axiom I, however, says nothing about similarity. And, for instance, to English ears, Finnish and Italian sound very similar, but are not related, whereas it would be hard to find two languages more dissimilar than the two related languages, English and Welsh. Again, the similarity both in sound and meaning might well lead the inquirer to suppose that Greek *hippos* "horse" and Danish *hoppe* "mare" were in some way connected. Axiom II, however, also says nothing about similarity, and these two words are in fact not connected. However, Modern English *warm*, Latin *formus*, Greek *thermós*, Sanskrit *gharmá-* are all congruent, despite the considerable difference in their initial consonant. And, to take an extreme example of dissimilarity, it is quite easy to demonstrate that *cow* and *beef* are really "one and the same word".

In conclusion, it may perhaps be observed that speech therapists may well find an especial interest in the question of how far the sound-changes of normal language may be paralleled in the speech of children and of those suffering from dyslalia, dysphasia and kindred disorders of speech. In Standard Spanish there has been a sound-change [z] > [ð], as in *plaza* "square", which is pronounced [plaða] – the change has not in general taken place in the Spanish of South America: this sound-change would appear to constitute a wholesale lisping!

6

G. PATRICK MEREDITH, Leeds

The Quantum of Language
— a psycho-physical interpretation
of the processes of communication

Dr Samuel Johnson once said "Men need to be reminded more often than they need to be informed". But we are all suffering today from a neurosis of novelty. This is the neurosis which the "hidden persuaders" have not failed to exploit. The talk which sells a product is the magic phrase "It's new!" This is also the neurosis of the millionaire. He delights not in his accumulation of wealth, nor in all that he could do with it, but only in its incessant augmentation. St Paul noticed the same neurosis in the Athenians, and in order to sell what he had to offer he had to appeal to their craving for novelty and to offer them "the unknown god".

Science today has the millionaire-neurosis. It allows its wealth of discovery to accumulate and delights only in adding to it. It is not the scientist who knows a great deal, but the scientist who has just made a new discovery, to whom we attend. And since neither the latter nor his listeners may make any attempt to relate the new discovery to the solid rock of previous knowledge, of which this novelty is but an outcrop, new discoveries are seldom seen in their true perspective. It is only when the rock threatens to topple over and bury us that we look beneath it and try to examine its foundations.

The rock of established science takes the form of a mountain of documents. I could give you figures to show the alarming rate at which this mountain is growing but you need only look in the periodical room of a library to see for yourself. Some scientists have developed an amusing defence-mechanism to protect them from the psychological menace of that mountain of unread literature, a formula which assures us that a scientific document has a life of only five years. After that it can be safely buried and forgotten. This formula is based on as neat a piece of circular reasoning as you will find in any textbook of logic. It was observed that the frequency with which old documents were consulted was much less than that for new documents. Ergo, old documents can be ignored because the majority of scientists seldom read them.

Now I am sure this insistence of mine on the importance of the past will seem very conservative and reactionary, and the idea that we have anything to learn from the past will be seen as the backward look of a fuddy-duddy. But genuine scientists do not ignore the past. The study of changes in rock-magnetism hundreds of millions of years back, for example, is vastly important in understanding the earth today. Likewise the steady accumulation of radio-active products which provides geologists, archaelogists and geo-physicists with their clock and time-scales, also serve to make the point. The point is that the past is not gone. It is with us still. It is a present reality. And being a reality it is active. It is this persistence of the past into the present which is one of the most essential principles to be grasped in seeking an understanding of the phenomena of language.

A student of language with no understanding of time is like a student of architecture with no understanding of space. The converse is also true, for architecture must reckon with time, and language occupies space as well as time. The Greeks went a long way in exploring the logic of space but they found time more resistant to their logic. Later through the discovery of perspective the laws of projection were elaborated and later still the non-quantitative relations of connexity, boundaries, neighbourhoods, overlaps, and so forth have given us a qualitative extension of geometry, namely topology. If we regard language as an attempt to map both the quantitative and the qualitative features of reality we see that all these geometrical concepts have an essential role to play in the analysis of language. Space remains an abstraction but the language of geometry enables us to clothe this abstraction in a gossamer garment of fine logic.

Time, too, is an abstraction, but by contrast with space it appears as a single line in which, given two events A and B, all we can say is either that A precedes B, or overlaps with B, or coincides with B, or follows B, and given any number of events we can arrange them according to these four relations. And these four relations are represented in the system of tenses of most Indo-European verbs. By contrast nouns do not normally have tenses, except by semantic implication as in such a word as "victim" or "residue". But we are all victims of circumstance and the material world of today is the residue of yesterday's events. The grammar which treats the noun as immune from the ravages of time, while making explicit the ephemeral character of the verb, foists on our minds a metaphysic which detaches matter from time and covers our linguistic map of reality with fictitious chasms unmatched in the real world.

Science has been busy pasting over these chasms by mathematical functions, by insisting, for example that particles are waves and vice versa, and that measurements of time are not independent of space, of velocity, of gravitational force and hence of matter. But as soon as the physicist steps out of his laboratory and uses everyday language he perforce becomes a metaphysician. And I have a notion that this incompatibility between the world as portrayed by physics and the world as pictured by everyday language is at the very fork of the divergence between the "two cultures" which C. P. Snow has diagnosed as the principal ailment of our civilization.

If I stress the importance of physics in seeking a fundamental understanding of the nature of language it is because alone among the sciences it has succeeded in breaking through the metaphysic of language. Biology, which should know better because it is so intimately concerned with mobile, developing tissues and labile substances, still separates anatomy from physiology, in other words space from time. And the amount of metaphysics packed into the prevailing terminology of psychology is enough to provide jobs for the disciples of Gilbert Ryle for generations to come. By contrast the engineers who understand the importance of fatigue in metals, of corrosion in pipes, of erosion in buildings, of subsidence due to mining, and the decay of nuclear products as well as the time required for engines to be "run in", reveal the craftsman's intuitive grasp of the logic of time.

To be fair to the biologists, they have shown us some of the laws of evolution, of heredity, of embryology and growth, all phenomena in which the logic of time is implicit. It is not their work but their language which needs scrutiny. And to make clear my position in stressing the importance of physics in the study of language this is not a claim that physics can supply all the answers. What physics has done is to show that matter is not made of tiny billiard balls but of systems of probabilities of events. Thus the syntactical unit of physical thought is neither the noun nor the verb but a union of the two. What physics still finds so resistant to explanation is the solid state, the seeming petrifaction of events which gives the visible world its rock-like stability and populates our grammar with nouns. Yet not only are all men mortal but even rocks decay and crumble, and the stars themselves have their births and deaths. Thus solid objects are but phases in an elongated system of events.

But these systems, which we call trees, men, stones, chairs, bacteria, planets and so on, are not isolated tracks in space-time. There is an endless traffic of events between them. We think of them as discrete objects only spasmodically involved with one another and independent betweenwhiles. But this is because our eyes dominate our brains. Philosophy and common-sense alike have been overwhelmingly shaped by the evidence of vision alone. Our ears and tongues and noses and skin and muscles, if we would heed them more often, would fill in many of the gaps left by vision. And if we had electromagnetic senses we should find the notion of independence hard to conceive. Through the instruments of physics we become aware of a continuum of forces stretching throughout all space to the most distant galaxy. The common-sense world of vision gives us fictitious islands in a continuous ocean of fact. But "fictitious" is too strong a word. They are fictitious only because we isolate them. In themselves, so long as we recognize their continuity of relationship, they are as real as the forces which relate them. And precisely because they are temporary stabilities in this ocean of changing forces we do well to moor our ships of exploratory thought to these comparatively fixed points.

Thus having demolished the noun as a metaphysical ultimate we must now rehabilitate it as a convenience of thought. It is like saying in mathematics "let A be a constant" and then for the duration of the theorem, however much x and y may vary, we know we can depend on A not to change because we have ordered it to stay put. And this is precisely what we attempt to do with words. We try to make them semantically invariant. We try to adopt dictionary definitions and to impose them on our children. The need for society to preserve its heritage of culture, as well as the daily need to refer verbally to common-sense objects, may be taken as the justification for this attempt at rigidity. Unfortunately words themselves seem to have a life of their own, and our attempts to freeze their meanings are continually thwarted. A word as a black mark on paper, with a definition attached, is like the constant A in a mathematical theorem. Regrettably the same word in its other manifestations refuses to obey our mathematical rules. The logician is continually defeated by the exuberant vitality of the living word.

Thus linguistics, to be true to the facts, must be more like biology than logic. We can only bring in logic at a different level – a level at which words as such have been analysed into systems of variables. The implication of this is that even the simplest word is far more complex than most linguists ever dreamed and that the practice of analysing words in terms of other words is simply to replace one complexity by another of the same kind. The more you analyse everyday words the more differences appear and instead of converging towards simplicity of explanation the philosophy of linguistic analysis leads to an ever-increasing complexity of argumentation. The followers of Wittgenstein behave like the sorcerer's apprentice, dealing with an endless splintering of splinters.

Let us note that chemistry could have gone the same way. If the chemists had tried to explain molecules in terms of molecules the subject would have remained bogged down in the confusion of alchemy. It was Dalton who first clearly discerned the essential methodological equation of chemistry, viz. that

$$\text{molecules} + \text{molecular laws} + \text{insight} \rightarrow \text{atoms}.$$

At a later stage the physicists applied the same equation to atoms and so arrived at the nucleus. This is not the end, of course. Every terminus in science is a new starting-point. But the laws of molecules and atoms still stand. They are not demolished by the laws of nuclei.

What kind of insight do we need to break through the everyday metaphysic of language, to discover its elements and the relations between them? Putting the question another way what are the true dimensions of language? In the theory of the chromatrope I have been attempting to define an element which requires a space of six dimensions for its complete representation. If you wish to represent a three-dimensional mountain on a flat map all you can do is to represent slices – contours and cross-sections. This works well enough so long as you bear in mind that by taking different intervals of measurement, and different directions for your sections, the results will appear different even though all represent the same mountain.

Each of these six dimensions represents a set of variables. These variables have only to be stated for it to be evident that they all enter into the determination of linguistic phenomena. Their grouping into six dimensions simply represents the fact that at present I see no way of reducing them to any lesser number if their essential characteristics are to be preserved. But this six-dimensional framework is not a metaphysical scheme of eternal categories. I prefer to call it an "interrogative framework". For its function is to enable us to ask systematic questions, to be answered by systematic experiment. These questions are of the following type: given any linguistic signal, which I shall call *sigma* (σ) what variables and what combinations of variables enter into its determination? With six sets of variables this requires us to seek answers to no less than 64 (i.e. 2^6) sets of questions. This at least should be a cure for dogmatism and will keep research-workers profitably occupied for years to come.

Picture a signal as a pulse of sound, a spherical zone of variations of atmospheric pressure, or of electromagnetic vibrations, or a letter in the mail. It has a starting-point and a destination. Work must be done to start it on its way, to preserve it from attrition, to deliver it safely, and it does work itself on arrival. The purely physical variables of energy-transformation involved in this aspect constitute what I call the Phi-dimension of language (ϕ).

Language has morphology. There is a pattern in the signal, a more or less elaborate geometrical structure either of graphic forms or of amplitudes and frequencies. These are not accidental forms out there in space. They are organized forms imposed by the muscles of the vocal organs or of the hand. The variables in this process of determining the organization of structure constitute the Beta-dimension (β).

In the use of language various objects and materials have to be controlled and set to work, such as pen, ink and paper, chalk and board, typewriter, microphone, lips, tongue and vocal chords, eyes and ears, wire and air. These all possess inertia, resistance and other measurable mechanical properties and many of them cost money. These material quantities, whether measured in terms of money, or human effort, or by physical instruments, necessarily enter into every act of communication. They constitute what I called the Theta-dimension (θ).

These three dimensions are recognizably physical, but if language is not a psycho-physical phenomenon I don't know what is. Hence my next three dimensions involve a reference to that four-letter word "mind", so shocking to the philosophers and the behaviourists. If they were as shocked by the word "matter" which is just as metaphysical as "mind" I could sympathize more with their Ockhamist scruples. As it is I shall go on being vulgar, using the word "mind" to refer to that more or less stable system of events which we describe by such terms as "experience", "communication" and "decision". These form the basis of my other three dimensions.

If we accept experience as the source of knowledge, and recognize that knowledge can vary in amount, any increase in knowledge being called "information", and if one, at any rate, of the primary functions of language is to communicate information, then we have a set of variables involved in such processes as perception, concept-formation, learning and memory, which all contribute to the mind's available store of information. In using language to communicate we draw upon this store. Thus it is one of the main determinants of our signals. This constitutes the Psi-dimension (ψ).

Communication is essentially a dyadic relation between a communicator and a recipient, an intimacy between two minds. If it is not this it is merely a curious fluctuation of energy. One has only to reflect on the stupendous consequences to which these fluctuations can give rise to recognize the triviality which so often appends the denigratory adjective "mere" to the noun "words". It is precisely because words establish an inter-personal relativity, an "I-thou" relation, and because so many of the world's events are incomprehensible apart from this relation, that we must recognize it as a dimension of mind. Between individuals it is a fluctuation of energy. Within the individual it is a human need, the need for human relationship, the hunger which binds societies. This constitutes the Lambda-dimension (λ).

Finally we have what some psychologists call "the decision-making mechanism". This is the source of selection, choice, novelty, creativity. We do not understand it. It baffles our expectations and plays havoc with our mathematical probabilities. It provides many of the mutations of personal development and of social evolution. Scientists tend to shy away from it because it spells unpredictability, but since they accept the unpredictability of decay in the individual atom why should they jib at the unpredictability of growth in the individual person? It is the variables of decision-making which constitute my sixth dimension, the Alpha-dimension (α).

Obviously these six dimensions need a lot of further elucidation but for our present purpose it suffices to say that they all add their characteristic quota of variation to the pattern of the signal. If we could measure all these variations, and determine their mathematical relationships as definite laws, the signal would be expressible as a single six-dimensional mathematical function. Let us call this function "the Signal Tensor". Now the interesting fact is that although we cannot yet determine the mathematical expression for this tensor our brains automatically solve the large numbers of equations required for each value of the tensor every time we speak to a friend or write a letter. I say "our brains" because most of these equations are solved without any conscious effort.

In the chromatrope theory I have tried to envisage a mechanism which would account for this extraordinary facility in solving large numbers of equations literally quicker than thought. In working out this mechanism I have been guided by three main concepts, viz. the *schema*, the mathematical *set*, and the *cell-assembly*. The concept of the schema has been developed by Head, Bartlett, Wolters, Zangwill, Oldfield, Vernon, Russell Brain and others. The *set* is the central concept in the foundations of mathematics due to Cantor. The *cell-assembly* is a powerful neurological concept principally due to Hebb. To these I have added the concepts of the Spectrum of Information, Semantic Matrices, Psycho-physical relativity and, my present topic, the Quantum of Language. To give formal definitions of all these would take too long and each depends on the others so that only in the chromatrope itself can their significance be seen.

I made mechanical models to emphasize that language-mechanisms, being manifestly located in brain-tissue, must be regarded as physical objects. Models are good servants but bad masters. If we try to use a mechanical model as, in itself, providing an explanation of some facet of human behaviour, we almost always fall into fallacy. Even the camera as a model for the eye does this. My only uses for models are to explore the physical implications of one's concepts and to force one to ask new questions. What the chromatrope theory says is that the philosophic contrast between *words* and *things* is as fallacious as the dualism of mind and body. Hence just as mind is incarnated and body is psychically organized in a continuum of psycho-physical processes, so also a *word* is a *thing* and we can make any *thing* to do the work of a word. A set of black marks on paper is indubitably a *thing* but so equally obviously is a set of cell-assemblies in the brain.

If by a "thing" we mean something hard, precisely localized and indifferent to the passage of time or to the existence of other *things*, then "things" are fictions. But in my sense of the word "thing" the members of the College of Speech Therapists constitute a thing. They are all professionally and historically related to a coherent stream of events, all (while living their variable lives) have something permanent in common, and all display psycho-physical properties. The Milky Way, in just the same sense, is a thing.

If now we regard a word in the brain as a *thing* in this sense, the concept at once forces us to ask – What are the components of this thing and do these components send signals to each other, as members of the College of Speech Therapists send letters to each other and stars send light to each other? And we at once realize that all the evidence of neurology, and particularly of aphasia, does indeed point to the conclusion that a word is a set of inter-communicating parts. So we next ask – What are the essential properties of these parts and how do they inter-communicate to create meaning, speech, writing, hearing and reading?

The answer which the chromatrope theory gives to this question is:

    1. that each brain possesses an individual *spectrum of information*, the product of countless acts of learning from infancy onwards, through all the senses and muscles;

2. that each little packet of learning, with its own fragment of the total spectrum, commands a distinct group of cells (possibly glia-cells as well as nerve-cells) not necessarily all adjacent but functioning as *collective unities*;

3. that each packet functions as an *information-resonator*, excited by any input of information whose spectrum overlaps with its own, and capable of exciting other packets by its characteristic radiation;

4. that groups of these packets function as *words* by reason of having been formed by many overlapping learning-processes in the past, and hence having more of the spectrum in common than any random collection of packets;

5. that because learning is a process which relates the organism to the environment while internally relating its experiences to each other, a word gains its unique power by being a *packet of relativity*;

6. that each individual performs millions of distinct acts of learning during his lifetime and hence possesses a large *statistical aggregate* of packets of learning organized into many thousands of words;

7. that the inter-radiations of the packets of learning constitute *word-formation*, and the inter-radiation of words constitutes *sentence-formation*;

8. that the total internal radiation at any moment constitutes the *mental set* which dominates interpretation, expression and attitude;

9. that the precise logical relations of the *mathematical sets* (using "set" quite differently here) provides the basis for the coherence and systematic functioning of language by determining the *patterns of resonance*;

10. that the collective public spectrum of information which constitutes our culture, while largely determining what individual spectra are possible, is only fractionally represented in the spectrum of any one individual, and hence *words never mean exactly the same to any two individuals.*

This commonplace fact of what may be called "semantic dispersion", so troublesome to lexicographers and logicians, thus receives a ready explanation in the chromatrope theory. Given the individuality of every mind it is, indeed, the amount of *convergence* of meaning that calls for explanation, rather than the divergence. Thermodynamics indicates a universal tendency towards disorder and randomization. Language is part of man's struggle in the other direction against the forces of chaos. But language, like any other behaviour, has to participate in the general physical flux of events. Its signals are pulses of radiation and their modes of determination must be interpreted in the light not only of the laws of thermodynamics but also of the laws of relativity.

But before discussing relativity I must revert for a moment to the aspect of time which physics so conspicuously neglects, viz. its *cumulativity*. By this I mean that aspect which forces itself on historians, on archaeologists, on evolutionary biologists, on geologists, and which should be of major concern to philologists and psychologists. It is largely ignored by physicists and chemists (except in such processes as photography) because they deal with theoretical particles devoid of memory. But at all grosser levels of magnitude both the ravages of time and the gains which its passage confers are universally in evidence. Thus the present properties and behaviour of every physical object above the molecular level require for their full interpretation an investigation of the past history of the object.

It follows from this that although the scientific observation of an object is a present event in the here and now, the signals which the body sends to our senses contain information, if we can but decipher it, concerning all its past history. When we see a man with a cauliflower ear and a flattened nose and say "he's a boxer" we are doing just this. And we can apply the same discernment to language.

The particulate character of language is a manifestation of the tendency of the continuum everywhere to condense into local or temporal singularities, and into systems of singularities. Every organism lives by establishing and varying an elaborate relativity with its surroundings. Among the latter are organisms of its own species. By reason of genetic and hence constitutional similarity the needs and experiences of organisms of the same species will all lie within a range different from the range of another species. Thus although the whole continuum is, by its nature, inter-communicating, the communications within a species allow of numerous highly specific correspondences. Near-identity of structure allows mutual resonance to occur. It is on this capacity for resonance that language-systems are built.

Every organism is both an energy-system and a relativity-system. It is a structure of cohesive forces which give it a certain variable stability from birth till death. Being finite its energy-transactions can vary only within a certain range. At fairly regular intervals there has to be an approximate balancing of the energy-budget. Competing with other organisms it has to develop principles of organic economy. The same principle of division of labour by which our industries have evolved has been at work for a thousand million years in organisms at all levels. The body of a plant or animal is an elaborate system of specialized cells, tissues and organs, each instrumental in performing a necessary function more economically than could a less specialized structure. The body is packed with natural patents which enable it to make enough profits to keep going.

These natural patents or instruments are, in fact, identical with the anatomy of the animal, but we grasp this equation only by viewing the whole anatomy functionally. This means recognizing every part as making a characteristic contribution to the economy of the organism. In establishing this equation we must also note that each organism, by reason of its ceaseless transactions with its environment, imposes modifications on the patents bequeathed to it by its ancestors. In other words it *learns*. Psychology treats learning as an important function, perhaps the most important function, but still a *function*, i.e. a process, an activity. This is correct as far as it goes but it is an activity which leaves a product behind it. What is so significant about this product is that *each specific case, when established, eliminates the need for the process by which it was produced.* By its subtle modification of the anatomical system it becomes itself a new anatomical device. As the eminent Russian psychologist Luria says (in *The Role of Speech in the Regulation of Normal and Abnormal Behaviour*, Pergamon Press, 1961):

"This process *creates a new information system within which each signal presented to the subject now operates.*"

I have made what may seem to be rather free use of the word "relativity" and to justify this I need the full force of that remark of Dr Johnson's with which I began this paper. Forty years ago I was just old enough to be affected by the immense intellectual excitement aroused by Einstein's theory, and just mathematical enough to start getting my teeth into its meaning. At that time the European heritage of coherent scientific thought, to which Germany, France and Britain had made the principal contributions, was still alive, though suffering from a mortal wound as a result of World War I. Today it is splintered into a thousand disconnected formulae, amenable to endless manipulations but with apparently little historic comprehension by their manipulators. The reminders of that heritage are beginning to appear, thanks to the stream of translations from the United States of the works of a handful of great German scientists and philosophers who struggled to safety and sanity. Austrians, Poles and Russians have likewise contributed to this material for a new Renaissance. Relativity must be seen in this perspective if its significance is to be grasped.

It is useless to try to understand the working of language in and between individuals unless we recognize that the language of each individual is a sample of his cultural heritage, and that every time he opens his mouth not only is his personal biography reasserting his personal past in the present moment, but the history of his people and of his neighbours is dominating the forms and consequences of his utterance.

In 1924 there appeared the English translation of Max Born's important and lucid exposition of Einstein's *Theory of Relativity* (published by Methuen). In a brief opening chapter he was able to put relativity in its cultural perspective in words which could scarcely be bettered today. And in the few sentences which time allows me to quote he pin-points the concept which is vital in our approach to man's present predicament, the split in our cultures and in the Cold War itself.

"The world" [he says] "is composed of the ego and the non-ego, the inner world and the outer world. The relations of these two poles are the object of every religion, of every philosophy. But the part that each doctrine assigns to the ego in the world is different. *The importance of the ego* in the world-picture seems to me a measure according to which we may order confessions of faith, philosophic systems, world views rooted in art or science, like pearls on a string.... All religions, philosophies and sciences have been evolved for the purpose of expanding the ego to the wider community that 'we' represent.... Einstein's theory... is a pure product of the striving after the liberation of the ego."

I cannot do justice to Max Born's insight here but is it not clear that the one thread that holds all these pearls together is language? And that in language alone are we to find the relations which stretch from pole to pole, the pole of absolute experience of the ego and the pole of metrical relations among physical objects. The current resistance of many humanists to physical concepts is due to an identification of physics with classical mechanics. And here I must quote from a contemporary of Max Born's, viz. Hans Reichenbach, who wrote in 1921 (English translation in *Modern Philosophy of Science*, 1959, Routledge and Kegan Paul):

"Classical physics and epistemology committed the error of regarding mechanical motion as the explanation of all phenomena. This was a prejudice because mechanics is not closer to the senses than optics and acoustics. Mechanics originated from the sense of touch, while optics was born of the sense of sight, and, in principle, it does not matter which kind of sense-perception physics takes as its starting-point. All those objections to the theory of relativity which charge it with being inconceivable arise merely because one is still preoccupied with a mechanical conception of the world; progress in science consists in overcoming mechanistic materialism, and the theory of relativity is the last great element in this development."

I have had to stress this rejection of mechanism because I used mechanical models myself in order to express my insistence on the principle that *words are things*. But if you study my model chromatropes you will find that the mechanism works by means of *light-signals* and this is far more essential to the concept than the model battleships which these signals set in motion, and which were shown at York to the British Association in 1959 (see "Models of Semantic Mechanisms", *Advancement of Science*, June 1960[1]). For although I insist that words are things I also insist that *language is radiation*.

[1] References appropriate to the present paper will be found in this article.

And hence whatever the theory of relativity says about radiation applies in principle to language. It was Einstein's insistence that our knowledge of mechanics is derived from *instruments*, i.e. clocks and measuring rods, and that the information we derive from these is by means of *light signals* travelling at a finite velocity, that undermined the Newtonian concepts of absolute space and time. The chromatrope theory treats the word-schemata in the brain as instruments. Each instrument receives and transmits information in the form of complex pulses of neural disturbance, each having its own characteristic spectrum. Radiation is simply a travelling disturbance of any kind, and though the medium of the brain is vastly more subtle than the field of interstellar space in which Einstein was primarily interested, and although we are dealing with pulsing bodies rather than moving bodies, these pulses are essentially light-signals and must obey the same laws.

What I mean by the "quantum of language" is the pulse of a chromatrope. And what I mean by a "chromatrope" is a packet of learning embodied in brain-tissue. The teeming population of chromatropes constitutes the assembly of instruments through which the ego negotiates its relations with other egos, and hence many of its relations with the physical world. In the complex spectra of these quanta, all biographically and historically determined, we can discern the iridescence of the pearls which Max Born saw as stretching from pole to pole. In the mutual resonance of these particles of learning we see the mechanism of the I-thou relation which gives the deepest meaning to our culture and civilization.

7

D. B. FRY, London

Coding and Decoding in Speech

If we pose the question: what is embodied in a man's speech? the only answer that seems to be sufficiently all-embracing is that it is his experience – experience which covers a long span of time, from his earliest moments as a human being to the few moments before he makes any particular utterance, experience which is of many different kinds, made up as it is of a life-time of instinctual, emotional and intellectual experiences. The question comes more sharply into focus, perhaps, when we imagine an individual speaker in a particular situation and ask what exactly will determine his next utterance, that is, what will decide what he says and the precise way in which he says it. His choice of words and phrases will depend very largely on his experience of the preceding seconds, on what he or someone else has just said. But it will depend too on his whole experience as a social animal, on his education and upbringing as well as on the needs of the moment. The actual speech-sounds that he produces, his pronunciation, will be partly a long-term product, affected by the speech of his parents, his school-fellows, the people he works with, and partly the result of the current situation, the general atmosphere, the person he is talking to, the need to talk quickly or slowly, loudly or softly. The rhythm and intonation of his speech will again be determined both by his background and by the situation and will contain an emotional component which is due to his reaction to the subject of conversation and to the people and things around him at the moment; the emotional reaction is itself a product of the speaker's personal psychology and history. Added to all this is the speaker's personal voice-quality which reflects many aspects of his personality, of his psychological and physiological condition, as well as being modified by the needs of the rôle that he is called upon to play in the particular situation.

All these kinds of information about an individual speaker are contained in his speech but it is given to few people, if indeed to any, to reach the speech of their fellow-men in such a variety of ways. In every feature of speech that has been mentioned, there is clearly a personal and a social component. The language learning process trains us all as speakers and listeners to take in most readily the content of speech which is due to social factors although we do, to a lesser extent, make use of the information that speech contains about the identity, the personality and the mood of the speaker. It is not surprising that this situation is somewhat paralleled with regard to scientific knowledge about speech; we know a great deal more about the social level of speech, that is about language systems and the way in which they are used, than we do about the manifestations of individual psychology in speech. Such things as voice quality, hesitation phenomena, certain aspects of rhythm and intonation, fall into the second category and are generally little understood. On the other hand, our knowledge of the ways in which linguistic information is transmitted, although very far from complete, is rapidly increasing.

The language code

The individual speaker whom we imagined ourselves observing in the act of utterance will speak in the virtual certainty of being understood; he will think of something to say, will say it and will expect that someone will know what he has said. This certainty, based naturally on previous experience, depends on the fact that he is using a code, that is a set of signals, restricted in number, whose use is governed by conventions. Communication by speech is possible only because all the signals are known to and the conventions agreed by the speaker and his hearers. This is in fact what we mean when we say that people have a common language, for all languages are codes, though of a very complex kind. Speakers and listeners are not usually aware that they are making use of a code; their knowledge of it is stored at a brain level where little attention is paid to it, but it remains true that language users must know the whole linguistic system and must abide by the conventions in using it if successful communication is to take place.

The most important feature of the code formed by a natural language, such as English, is that it is a hierarchical system, a system consisting of several levels and organized in such a way that units which function on one level combine to form the units on the level next above. The English language code, for example, comprises four levels; the units at the lowest level are the phonemes which combine together to form the units at the next level, the morphemes, which have grammatical function; morphemes joined together form words, which have lexical function, and words combine to form sentences. The speaker and listener who use this code must know both the different units that can occur and also the rules according to which the units on one level combine to form units on the next level. At the lowest level, the phonemic level, the total number of different units is relatively small; the English phonemic repertory contains about forty items. As soon as we move to the next level, the morphemic, the number of possible units is very much greater; the forty English phonemes in combination provide many thousands of morphemes and words and these in turn can be arranged in an even larger number of possible sentences. It is worth noticing that an individual speaker does not add to his phonemic repertory (within his native language) after he has learned to talk. By the age of five or seven years the child generally has the phonemic system complete and does not add to it throughout the rest of his life. This is in contrast with the other levels of the code, for he is likely to be learning new words and hence acquiring the capacity to form new sentences for many years. But whatever fresh morphemes or words the speaker may acquire, they will not contravene the laws that govern the combination of phonemes in the particular language; an Englishman may at some stage add the word *parasitology* to his word inventory but not a word /pwarasitolədʒi/ since the sequence /pw/ in word-initial position is not allowed by the English code. This is an example of the kind of information which all language users have, although they are quite unaware of it, and, as we shall see later, they know not only what is possible or impossible but also what is probable or improbable in a given context.

Knowledge of the code, of the levels, the possible units and the laws of combination is stored in the brain of every speaker and listener. The speaker who is about to utter must first of all organize what he is going to say in its appropriate coded form. This means that at some cortical level he formulates what he has to say in sentences which are made up of appropriate words, each consisting of the required morphemes, each morpheme being a sequence of phonemes. Not much is yet known about the encoding process in the speaker but from evidence that will be touched upon a little later it is clear that in spontaneous speech a speaker does not formulate a complete sentence before he begins to speak; he is as it were improvising from moment to moment. Hence encoding is a continuing process during speech. It is not, however, a continuous process for it goes forward generally in little spurts. In any sentence there are some words whose function is to determine the grammatical shape of the sentence – the *form* words – and yet others which largely determine the content of the sentence – the *content* words. Before he begins a sentence, the speaker generally has some idea of the form of the sentence he is going to utter and also of its content. During the encoding, however, form words are more readily found and organized in sequence than content words and hence there is a tendency for encoding to proceed rapidly through sequences of form words and to slow down or to stop at the points where there are content words.

This view of language coding by the speaker is based largely on the results of experimental work by Dr Goldman-Eisler who has made an extensive study of hesitation phenomena in speech. Two kinds of pauses occur in speech – those which are imposed by the need for inspiration and those which are the result of hesitation on the part of the speaker. The incidence of breath pauses in normal speech, whether it be spontaneous speech, reading from a text or repeating by heart, is determined by the syntax of the language. The speaker will pause for breath at points in the sequence where some syntactical unit is complete, at the end of a sentence, a clause or a phrase, in fact at places where in a text there would generally be some mark of punctuation. In spontaneous speech there are always, in addition to breath pauses, interruptions of the sequence by hesitation, even in the case of the most fluent speakers. Dr Eisler's work has shown that the occurrence of hesitation pauses and indeed their actual duration are a function of the flow of information during speech. Information is used here with the sense which it has in information theory, that is to say it is equivalent to predictability.

Any word in a sequence which is highly predictable supplies very little information whereas words which are not predictable convey a great deal of information. In this sense form words contain relatively little information since most of them can be predicted with ease; content words as a class carry more information and vary considerably in their predictability. The experiments reported by Dr Eisler show that speakers tend to pause before words whose information content is high and the duration of the pause is correlated with the predictability of the word which follows the pause. This indicates that in the encoding process the speaker's brain requires a longer time to select the more unusual words but produces the more common words, and particularly the form words, rapidly and without hesitation. This suggests that the length of the unit encoded at this level is dependent on the information rate and may be approximately one content word with the ensuing form words.

It should be stressed here that the encoding process at this stage is a form of cortical activity, that is to say it consists of patterns of nerve impulses and connections. The code we are discussing is therefore, from one point of view, a neural code. The relation of this to the language code can perhaps be best understood by using the analogy of the Morse code. The dots, dashes and spaces of the latter are independent in one sense of the particular language (English, French, German, etc.) for which the code is used and yet they provide a form in which the sentences and words of these languages can be stored and transmitted. In a somewhat similar way, the nerve impulses of the neural code are a form in which the language code of English, for example, can be stored and used in the brain of an English speaker. The memory stores required for communication by speech can be thought of as a very large number of neural circuits in the brain bearing coded signals which are available to the speaker and the listener when they need them. The encoding process consists in drawing from the store the right signals in the right order and using them to control the next stage of the speech process, the action of the muscles.

The control system

The function of the brain in the coding process is twofold: it selects the language units and arranges them in the appropriate order and provides a flow of operating instructions to be transmitted along neural pathways to the sets of muscles involved in speech. The second of these functions is as complex as the first. It consists in the transformation, the re-coding in effect, of the message from its linguistic form into terms of respiratory, laryngeal and articulatory muscle activity. The rhythm of quiet breathing is changed, the expiratory phase is very much lengthened and the moment of inspiration is dictated by the grammatical form of the message. During expiration the rate of air-flow is continuously controlled and at the same time the chest muscles are used to impart the syllabic structure to the utterance. The laryngeal muscles receive their instructions not only in accordance with the successive voiced or unvoiced nature of the sounds demanded by the phoneme sequence but also as a result of the emotional factors which are mediated by the brain and which affect both the variations in larynx frequency and the tensions in the muscles which influence voice quality. In addition there is the articulatory action of the muscles of the pharynx, the tongue, the soft palate and the lips which is the principal correlate of the phonemic sequence.

This manifold muscular activity is finely co-ordinated and controlled by the brain; the relative timing of the action of different muscles is determined within very close limits. The required degree of control is achieved by the use of feed-back circuits in addition to the feeding forward of instructions to the muscles. All the time that the skilled movements of speech are being made, the brain of the speaker is receiving information through the auditory, kinaesthetic and tactual feed-back loops about the progress of the movements. This information is of primary importance for the timing and co-ordination of the various components in the complex patterns of muscular activity as we can see from the dramatic disruption of speech which usually results from delayed auditory feed-back.

The action of linguistic coding that has already been mentioned produces as it were a programme which it is the task of the control system to implement. The control system works in the neural code, that is the "on-or-off" language of the nerve impulse, but the complete pattern of nerve activity for a single utterance or even for part of an utterance is of tremendous complexity. Further, different parts of the system may deal with different time-spans: the neural control of variation in vocal cord frequency may, for example, be programmed for a complete phrase or even a sentence at a time while articulation is programmed for considerably shorter stretches. In the case of articulatory movements there are some grounds for thinking that the unit length for control patterns is about that of the syllable, that is to say that the whole sequence of articulatory movements for one syllable is programmed at one time. A speaker who corrects an error in his articulation does not usually do so in mid-syllable; he has at least to wait until the syllable is finished before he goes back to make the correction (though he may wait very much longer than this). There may also be some significance in the fact that delayed auditory feed-back has the maximum effect on most speakers when the delay is something a little less than the average duration of a syllable.

If we review the coding process so far as we have examined it, we see that during an utterance the speaker's brain must first carry out the linguistic encoding, which it will probably do for a few words at a time in spontaneous speech. As a result there is a very complex transmission of neural signals in the control system, to the respiratory muscles both to determine the moments of inspiration and to govern the rhythmic structure of the speech, to the laryngeal muscles to control voice quality, vocal cord frequency and the on-off switching of voice demanded by the phonemic sequence and to the muscles used in articulation in order to produce the movements appropriate to the phoneme sequence in the particular language that the speaker is using.

The articulatory code

The purpose of the control signals, as we have said, is to produce the skilled movements of speech. At this point the form of the message changes into patterns of activity on the part of many different sets of muscles. Although these muscles are concerned with respiration and phonation as well as with articulation, it will be convenient to think of the message at this stage as being formulated in the *articulatory code*, since articulation is indispensable to any utterance which is related to a language system.

When the message is transformed into the articulatory code an important change takes place. Up to this moment the coding of the message has been in terms of signals which are clearly discrete. Both in the case of the units which make up the linguistic code and in the all-or-none signals of the neural control code, we are dealing with events which are either present or absent; we are not faced with things which happen more or less nor with classes which shade into each other without a clear boundary between one class and the next. The movements of speech are, however, continuous in time during a single utterance; further, they are composed of interwoven patterns of movement on the part of different sets of muscles, laryngeal, pharyngeal, tongue, soft palate and facial muscles. Even if we could obtain a complete record of this complex of movements for an utterance, it would not be possible to segment the record, to make cuts at two points on the time scale and say that the section between these points constitutes a given item in the code. It is meaningful to speak of an articulatory code only in the sense that movements can be placed qualitatively in different categories which represent, as it were, a projection of the linguistic code. The phonetic classes into which the movements of articulation are sorted are the counterpart of the phonemic level in the language code and are useful just because they enable us to see how the oppositions implied in the phonemic system are embodied in movement. The opposition of English /p/ and /k/ is realized in the articulatory code by the difference between a bi-labial and a velar movement; the opposition /t : s/ by the difference between an alveolar stop-release and an alveolar fricative signal; the opposition /n : d/ by the difference between a nasal continuant and an oral stop-release signal and so on. The articulatory code for the speakers of a given language will contain as many terms as the phonemic system requires. Since phonemic codes are different in different languages, it follows that the articulatory codes must also differ. English speakers, for example, differentiate between an alveolar fricative movement in *save* and a post-alveolar fricative movement in *shave*. In languages such as Dutch and Spanish where this opposition does not exist in the phonemic system, there is a corresponding absence of differentiation in articulation and consequently a wider variation from speaker to speaker in the articulations for /s/.

The signals of the articulatory code in a particular language are determined therefore by what is significant in that language. We have spoken so far only of movements that affect sound quality but the same thing is true of the muscle actions which realize rhythmic and intonation patterns; the movements embody all the significant features of rhythm and intonation. Speech movements, however, inevitably contain a great deal besides what is significant. A man's trousers flap when he is walking but from the point of view of getting from place to place there is nothing very significant about trouser flapping. In the same way, movements which are essential for a particular articulatory signal give rise to concomitant movements which are irrelevant from the point of view of the code. Further, since speech movements are continuous, many features of the total movement for an utterance are the effect of the order in which the various movements have to be made. The situation here is rather analogous to that of hand-writing; the muscular movements in writing embody, for everyday purposes, a code containing fifty-two letters, ten figures and several punctuation marks (including wordspace). When the movements are strung together, the resulting manuscript shows many features which are irrelevant from the point of view of the code and are due partly to the individual style of the writer and partly to interaction between the various movements. The result, as in speech, is a number of continuous patterns which embody the signals of the code but which also contain many irrelevant features and many variations of form which are brought about by the continuous nature of the movements. We shall see later why it is possible in the case of both speech and hand-writing to read such signals with comparative ease despite the extreme variability of the forms encountered.

The acoustic code

The sound-waves of speech represent the last transformation in the transmission phase of speech communication. The speech movements impose minute pressure changes on the expired air and these are propagated in all directions as sound-waves. The correspondence between the movements and the sound-waves is very close; that is to say that any change in the conformation of the vocal tract will entail a corresponding change in the wave-form of the sound issuing from the speaker. It follows therefore that just as the movements for an utterance are continuous so the wave-form of the sound is continuous, and hence it presents the same difficulties in the matter of segmentation. The simplest acoustic description of an utterance is provided by the wave-form, which is a graph of the amplitude of displacement of an air particle in the path of the wave at successive moments in time. Such curves are given by the oscillograms of speech commonly shown on a cathode-ray oscillograph. The oscillogram of an utterance shows that the sound-wave varies continuously throughout the utterance and it is not possible to cut up the wave into segments, each of which corresponds to a single muscular movement. The acoustic coding of the message therefore has this in common with the articulatory coding, that the signals are realized in forms which evince great variability owing to interaction between different stretches of the wave and to individual differences between speakers.

In order to arrive at the acoustic code we need to be able to separate out what is significant from what is irrelevant in the acoustic signals just as we needed to do for the articulatory code. There are two ways in which this task might be approached: the first is by looking in the acoustic sphere for features which correspond to significant articulatory differences, that is to say by seeking some acoustic feature that is present whenever there is a bi-labial articulation, a fricative articulation, a lenis articulation and so on. The second is to try to discover what acoustic features are significant for the listener, that is to say for the reception phase of speech communication.

For either method the simple account of the sound wave in terms of amplitude variation with time, that is the wave-form, is not very suitable and has to be replaced by some more analytical description. This is generally given by measurements of the distribution of energy throughout the frequency range coupled with measurements of the total sound intensity and of the fundamental frequency, and by the variation of all these quantities with time. Information of this kind is supplied by the various sound spectrographs which in recent years have become very widely used as a means of presenting acoustic data concerning speech.

Much of the spectrographic work on speech that has been done has been designed to discover the acoustic code by the first of the methods mentioned above. This has led to only partial success because the amount of information contained in the speech sound-waves is greatly in excess of that required for the understanding of speech – the proportion of irrelevant to significant information in other words is high – and also because the reception of speech depends upon relative and not upon absolute differences. Here once more the code is based on oppositions, on the fact that signal a is not signals b, c or d, and the means by which these oppositions are carried, as we shall see in the next section, differs in different contexts and conditions.

Most of what we know about the acoustic code has in fact been derived by the second method, that of discovering what acoustic features are significant for the listener. These features are, of course, expressed in terms of spectral distribution of energy, fundamental frequency, over-all intensity and time, and the only certain way of finding out what aspects of the acoustic pattern are significant is by making systematic variations in these dimensions and noting listeners' reactions to the changes. Synthetic speech, that is artificially produced speech-like sounds in which all the dimensions can be controlled, has been widely used for this purpose and these experiments have yielded a great deal of valuable information about the acoustic code in English, for example. In examining the acoustic signals from the point of view of their significance for the listener we are, however, no longer dealing with the encoding aspect of speech but with the decoding process, and it will be well therefore to go on to a consideration of decoding since this will itself necessitate an account of the acoustic code.

The decoding process

We have reviewed very briefly the stages by which the language units selected and arranged in the speaker's brain are coded and re-coded in various forms until the message emerges eventually in the form of sound-waves. The sound-waves reach the ear of the listener and the process of decoding consists in the operations that have to take place in order that the listener's brain may recover or reconstruct the sequence of language units in which the message was originally formulated.

Each stage of the encoding process has its counterpart in decoding. The speech sound-waves arrive first at the ear of the listener where they give rise to mechanical movements on the part of the ear-drum, the ossicles of the middle-ear, the fluids and hair-cells of the inner ear. It is a matter of some importance that these movements are mechanical in contrast to the skilled movements of the vocal tract in the encoding operation. No learning takes place in the peripheral hearing mechanism. The sound-waves are transformed by the ear in certain respects, with regard to frequency and intensity, but these changes are beyond the control of the listener and cannot be influenced by learning. The movements of the ear mechanism are converted into a neural code by the auditory nerves and it is these neural signals that are finally decoded as language units by the listener's brain. As we have seen, the acoustic wave is continuous but it is converted into discrete signals by the all-or-none nature of the nerve impulses.

The ability of the brain to decode speech is entirely the result of learning. We have noted already that a speaker and a listener can talk to each other only if they have a common language, that is if both brains hold a store of common information about a particular language system. If this is not the case, no communication takes place. Let us imagine a speech being given, say, in the Cantonese dialect of Chinese; in the audience next to each other are a listener who knows the language and another who does not. The same sound waves are arriving at the ears of both, the mechanical ear movements are the same for both, nerve impulses in the auditory nerves are the same in both and yet one is able to decode the speech and the other is quite unable to do so. This example stresses the paramount importance for decoding of the information stored at the centre. The reception of speech is a function both of what comes in and of what is already stored in the system; the force of the latter is such that if there is conflict between the signals perceived and knowledge already stored in the brain the conflict is most often resolved in favour of the latter and in contradiction to the signals that have come in.

The acoustic signals which arrive at the ear of the listener and are converted into neural signals give rise in the brain to patterns which correspond to percepts. The physical dimensions of the speech sound-waves, frequency, intensity and duration, have been replaced by perceptual dimensions, quality, pitch, loudness and length. The first operation on the part of the central decoding mechanism is to sort these perceptual patterns into the lowest level of language units, the phonemes. A number of general features of the decoding mechanism are involved in this operation and it will be as well to consider these in some detail before going on to the succeeding stages of decoding.

The scanning operation

We are dealing here with a process of recognition: a certain pattern has come into the system and it is necessary for decoding to identify this pattern as belonging to a certain class. If one wished to carry out a similar operation in a machine one would use some method of pattern-matching. The machine would have to contain a store of patterns representing all the classes into which the incoming patterns were to be sorted; then, when a fresh pattern was fed into the machine the store would be "scanned", that is the incoming pattern would be compared in turn with the stored patterns until it was found to match one of the latter; it would then be labelled as belonging to this class. There can be little doubt that in recognizing perceived patterns of many different kinds the brain acts in this way, with the important difference that it seldom needs to scan the complete repertory of patterns of one kind; it is able on the basis of past experience to narrow the field of stored patterns that must be scanned to a small proportion of the total.

The brain mechanism to deal with the phonemic level of English, for example, would need to sort incoming patterns into forty classes or categories. We can think of the scanning operation as being carried out in one of two ways: either there are a considerable number of different patterns associated with each phonemic category and the incoming pattern is put into a given category if it matches any one of the patterns stored in that class, or else each category is represented by a single pattern which has a complex of significant features, and in this case an incoming pattern is placed in a given category if it forms a sufficiently good match with the "master" pattern for that class. We might visualize the scanning device as being rather analogous to the "pattern-matching" toys that are often given to very young children and which consist of a container with a number of different shaped slots in its lid into which objects of various shapes have to be "posted". Each object can be put into the container only through the right slot. In the case of the phonemic scanner, the container would be divided into forty separate compartments. If we take the first view mentioned above, then the lid over each compartment would contain a number of differently shaped slots and quite a range of incoming patterns would enter the compartment through the slots which they matched. On the second view, the lid of each compartment would have one very complex slot through which would pass any pattern whose features formed a close enough match with the slot. The slots for all the phonemic compartments would be different and each would admit only the appropriate range of incoming patterns.

The classifying of incoming speech sounds into phonemic categories by such a pattern-matching technique is clearly only the very first stage in the decoding process. It is the only point at which decoding depends on the acoustic code and it forms a small part of the total operation of speech reception. The experiments with synthesized speech referred to above have produced a good deal of information about the acoustic code for English and have revealed a number of facts about the general nature of this part of the decoding process, which we may conveniently call "primary recognition".

Primary recognition

This refers specifically to the phonemic classification of incoming sounds by the listener on the basis of acoustic features and with the minimum of help from context, the kind of recognition we rely on when we hear for the first time an unusual proper name such as, for example, Slaithwaite. An English listener would have no difficulty in recognizing this phonemic sequence as /sleiθweit/ and he would do so by means of this knowledge of the acoustic code.

We cannot yet give a full account of the acoustic code for any language and it will in any case be possible to give here only a general idea of the way in which primary recognition works for English. We have already seen that phonemic classification is a matter of oppositions; the first important fact about primary recognition is that there are always several acoustic cues available for establishing a given opposition. The second important fact is that acoustic cues consist in relations between physical quantities and not in absolute values.

The long-established formant theory of vowel recognition exemplifies these properties of the acoustic code. The pure vowels of English constitute a system determined acoustically by the frequency of Formant 1, the frequency of Formant 2, the interval between these two frequencies, the interval between the fundamental frequency and that of Formant 1, the relative intensities of Formant 1 and Formant 2 and the fundamental. All these cues can be used by the listener to decide which member of the system is represented by a particular incoming signal but generally only a selection of them will be used by the listener at one time, that is in one set of conditions or in one context. Furthermore, the vowels form a system in which the relations between members are the important factors. Thus the quantities expressing the formant frequencies and intensities for the vowels spoken by a child are different, on an absolute scale, from those of the vowels spoken by an adult, yet, within each system, the listener has no difficulty in decoding the vowel signals. It can be shown experimentally that, on the other hand, changing the relationship of formant frequencies artificially can alter the place of vowels within the system.

Other features of the acoustic code for English have been disclosed by experiments on the recognition of consonants of various kinds. The cues used for decoding the voiceless plosives, /p, t, k/, have been shown to be mainly the frequency of the burst of noise produced by the release of the stop and the change in frequency (the transition) of the second formant of the periodic sound which precedes or follows the release.

The opposition between the fortis and the lenis consonants is signalled in a variety of ways in the acoustic code; it may depend on the presence or absence of a low frequency component resulting from vocal cord vibration, on the relative duration of the consonant wave-form and that of an associated periodic sound or on the fact that Formant 1 begins late in the adjoining periodic sound after a fortis initial consonant and ends early before a final fortis consonant.

For fricative consonants, again, the signal pattern in the acoustic code contains a number of features. If we take only the fortis fricatives, /θ, f, s, ʃ/, we find that the /s : ʃ/ distinction depends largely on a difference in spectrum, /s/ showing a peak higher in the frequency range than /ʃ/; /θ/ and /f/ together are opposed to /s/ and

/ʃ/ by having much less over-all intensity and /θ/ differs from /f/ in the second formant transition of the associated periodic sound.

Primary recognition then is the decoding of the acoustic code by matching patterns whose features are of the kind we have just outlined. The result of this first decoding operation is a sequence of phonemic units which form the basis for the succeeding stages of decoding. It order to understand these later stages we must now consider what is by far the most important factor in the whole process of the reception of speech.

The role of redundancy

This factor can be summed up by saying that no one would ever understand speech at all if he did not know what to expect. At any point in a message, what has gone before determines to a greater or less degree what may follow and this holds good at every level, the phonemic, morphemic, word and sentence levels in the linguistic code and equally in the neural, articulatory and acoustic codes. This feature of speech is referred to technically as the redundancy of speech; it means that everything in speech is to some extent predictable. If a signal is predictable then at least some of the information contained in the signal itself is not absolutely necessary for its decoding. There is therefore some connection between the technical sense of redundancy and the everyday use of the word. When decoding speech, the listener always has more information available than he needs.

We said earlier that in order to communicate by speech both speaker and listener must know the language system, which includes the phonemic system. Every signal that comes in must be one of the forty phonemes, in English, and not something outside the system. Recent experiments have shown that the actual perception of speech sounds is the result of the language learning process. When we learn our native language our perceptions are so trained and modified as to facilitate the phonemic grouping of incoming speech sounds.

In the reception of speech, primary recognition serves only to provide as it were the scaffolding on which is built the phonemic sequence for in addition to its ability to transform the acoustic code, the listener's brain has also an extensive knowledge of the statistics of phoneme occurrence. Thus at any point in the message it knows what are the probabilities that the succeeding phoneme will be phoneme x or phoneme y; this is true for the first position in a message as well as for other positions for certain phonemes and phoneme sequences are more probable at the beginning of an utterance than are others. It can be shown by experiment that in decoding current speech a listener can guess up to about 50% of the phonemes occurring in a sequence. This explains why, despite the great variability of the acoustic signals of speech, as also of the visual signals in hand-writing, we are able to decode both systems with ease.

The first stage of the decoding process, which consists in getting from the sound-waves of speech to the phonemic sequence, is effected therefore by combining the decoding of the acoustic code with the knowledge of phoneme statistics which every listener carries in his brain as a result of his experience in dealing with the language. All that has been said about phonemic decoding is equally applicable to the decoding of rhythmic and intonation features. There are acoustic cues for both which provide a basis for primary recognition and in addition there is some degree of redundancy which allows the listener to use his ability to predict the probable course of a rhythmic or intonation pattern.

Morpheme, word and sentence decoding

It is important to realize that perception of speech sound-waves plays a part only in the stage of primary recognition. All succeeding stages of decoding depend entirely on knowledge of the language system and language statistics. The phoneme sequence is arrived at by the scanning process already described and forms the input for the next operation which is the combining of phonemic units into morphemes. This requires the same kind of scanning process as before but the reference patterns are now morphemes and the incoming patterns are phoneme sequences. When the latter have been identified as morphemes, the next stage of decoding takes place which compares combinations of morphemes with stored words and in the subsequent stages, word sequences are matched with stored sentences which form the end result of the decoding process.

At all levels after the phonemic, the only criteria which are applied are (1) Is the decoded signal a possible one, that is to say, is it a possible morpheme, a possible word or sentence in the language? and (2) Does it fit in with what has gone before? The effects of what has preceded are often referred to as the constraints which govern the sequence and each level has its own constraints. When the listener is scanning morphemes to find a match for an incoming phoneme sequence, then morphemic constraints operate. A match may be found which is a possible morpheme in the language but it may be one which goes against the morphemic constraints in the particular context. This situation brings into play one of the most important features of the whole speech decoding mechanism, the very great capacity which it embodies for error correcting. If the particular morpheme were very unlikely this information would be fed back to the phoneme level and as a result an error might be corrected. The decision might be, for example: the phoneme which was recognized as /s/ should have been decoded as /θ/ and the morpheme is not *sink* but *think*, which fits in with the morphemic constraints. This type of error correction happens continually in the reception of speech and is the reason why it is necessary to postulate the serial decoding process that has been outlined here. Every scanning level is connected with those below so that such corrections can be made and further the output of each stage is held in the memory for some time so that, for example, sentence constraints may cause the listener to correct a phonemic or morphemic error which occurred even in a previous sentence. It may be noted in passing that these connections between levels are important also for the correction of errors which occur during the encoding of the message; they provide the mechanism which enables the speaker to go back and correct himself.

It must be stressed again in conclusion that all these operations are carried out at a brain level where both speaker and listener are generally unaware of what is happening (although error correction sometimes makes them temporarily more aware). In everyday language we simply say that we are able to take in speech because we know what it "means", but if we examine closely what this implies it becomes clear that from one point of view "what it means" is precisely an expression of all the constraints which operate in a given situation and at all levels.

8

JOHN R. BROOK, Maidstone

Aids to Diagnosis and Therapy

The place of speech therapy among the sciences has been pointed out by Dr Stein in Chapter 2. The student of speech therapy studies anatomy, psychology, neurology, phonetics, physics of sound and many other subjects. It would seem that while the specialist learns more and more about less and less, the speech therapist is obliged to learn more and more about more and more.

Borrowing a number of unrelated facts from other disciplines will not be of any lasting help to us. It is essential that we understand the facts we acquire and how the worker has arrived at his conclusions.

An increasing number of machines, especially of the electronic variety, are being used to aid observation and experiment; in order to understand and make use of results it is necessary to understand the equipment. In undertaking our own research we need to make use of all the applicable tools that modern technology can place at our disposal; for greater consistency and precision in diagnosis we must use as many means as we can. In fact, we must move with the times and if the times give us tape recorders, oscilloscopes and audio-analysers we should look carefully to see if we can use them.

Some time ago I asked Dr Stein why there is so much controversy among speech therapists over terminology. With typical forthrightness he answered that it is because we do not know what we are talking about. With instruments that record, measure and analyse, precisely and accurately, defective as well as so-called normal speech sounds we can undertake research, substantiate what we are talking about and perhaps add a little to the understanding of speech and language.

Most clinics now have tape recorders, but it is possible that many speech therapists know little about the relative usefulness of the many different makes, as applied to their particular needs.

Another piece of equipment with which speech therapists are relatively familiar is the audiometer. The Peters SPD/5 is an advanced clinic audiometer with which a very wide range of pure tone and speech tests can be applied. There are two continuously variable attenuators each readable and accurate to less than one db. A narrow band of white noise is available which automatically follows the tone frequency or the full white noise spectrum can be used. The noise can be put to the ear not being tested or can be mixed with this signal. The frequency is continuously variable from 125 to 12000 c/s for air and 250 to 8000 c/s for bone conduction. It is claimed to be very stable and accurate. There is automatic interruption or modulation of the tone. These together with many other features make this a most comprehensive audiometer.

Amplivox have an interesting portable audiometer. This is the model 51 which is independent of mains supply and weighs only 7 lbs 6 ozs with the carrying case and the headset. There are nine fixed frequencies from 250 to 8000 c/s for air conduction only. Amplivox also produce a clinical audiometer. This is the model 82 and has ten fixed air conduction frequencies from 125 to 8000 c/s and seven for bone conduction from 250 to 4000 c/s. Intensity level is in 5 db steps and a second channel is available for loudness balance tests. Narrow band masking may be automatically selected for each frequency from 250 to 4000 c/s. There is also a speech circuit. The Amplivox speech audiometer is basically a battery-driven gramophone with a calibrated transistor amplifier.

Both Amplivox and Multitone supply auditory training equipment. The Multitone equipment is for use with either an induction loop or with a headset for one child. The Amplivox apparatus may also be used for an induction loop or with headsets up to twelve in number, these usually being fitted to desk control boxes.

Cunningham Beattie of London produce a throat microphone. This microphone is held in position against the speaker's larynx by a light steel band. It is sensitive only to the mechanical vibrations of the larynx and not to the noise of the surroundings. The microphone is being developed for various applications and Cunningham Beattie are hoping to combine it with a transistorized amplifier to be worn on the chest. They would like to make contact with any therapists who work with patients who might be helped by such an aid. It is suggested that the patient with a weak voice due to a neurogenic condition might benefit or possibly the laryngectomized patient who can use pseudo-voice, but cannot produce enough volume of sound in some conditions.

Dawe Instruments make three pieces of equipment of interest to the speech therapist. (1) The audio analyser is intended for measurement of the relative amplitude of the component frequencies of a sound wave; thus it could be used to analyse a speech sound. For instance we are told that the mongol often has a low hoarse voice. With an analyser it would be possible to measure the difference between the mongol's voice and the normal voice rather than roughly estimating it by ear. (2) The sound level meter, used in conjunction with the analyser, measures the level or volume of a sound. These are sometimes used in conjunction with free field audiometry to estimate the level of sound being received by the patient. (3) The stroboscope is basically an instrument for producing a rapidly flashing beam of light. When oscillating objects such as the vocal folds are viewed in this light the movements seem to be slowed or stopped. Thus the stroboscope is used to view the vocal folds in motion.

The output of the analyser is displayed on a Cossor oscilloscope. This has an immense number of applications and is a very valuable teaching device. It has the attraction of looking remarkably like television (and I think the programmes compare well). It can be used to show a picture of a sound wave or electrical wave, etc., as the phenomenon occurs. It therefore has obvious advantages over the blackboard and cardboard model approach to the teaching of the fundamentals of sound and so on.

Two pieces of apparatus which are of great interest to the speech therapist have been designed in the Phonetics Laboratory of the University of London, which is under the direction of Professor D. B. Fry. The first demonstrates delayed auditory feedback, the second is a sound spectrograph.

This apparatus, like the Dawe analyser, tells us the relative level of the component frequencies in a sound. It produces the result, however, as a picture of the sound on an oscilloscope screen. Thus we have a picture of the sound as it occurs. This could obviously be used to examine and compare the defective speech sounds of, for instance, a group of dyslalic patients.

Apparatus which contrasts with the others in that it is not driven by electricity is the test for phenylketonuria by Ames. I think that there are an increasing number of patients with this condition coming to the attention of the speech therapist.

I should like to thank the manufacturers for their help. I am sure that anyone who approaches them with any problems will be met with the greatest cooperation.

9

JOAN H. van THAL, London

Evaluating the Nature and Degree of Defects and Disorders of Voice, Speech and Language

Effects are correlated with causes. Appropriate treatment for those suffering from disorders of communication demands investigation of the cause and careful scrutiny of the effect. The recognition of such causes is partly a medical function. Speech therapists have the necessary *"expertise"* for evaluating the defects of voice, speech and language due to factors other than signs and symptoms as defined in medical terminology.

Webster's International Dictionary gives the following definitions of the word "diagnosis":

"(1) (*Medical*) The art and act of recognizing the presence of disease from its signs and symptoms and deciding its character. (2) Scientific determination of any kind. (3) (*Botany and zoology*) A concise technical description of a species or group, giving the distinguishing character. (4) General perception and scrutiny; judgement based on scrutiny."

Thus diagnosis is not solely a medical term; the fourth definition applies very aptly to logopedics and so, to some extent, does the second. There is, therefore, a logical argument for the use of this word by speech therapists; objections to its use seem to be tinged with emotion and are not purely logical.

Even in highly cultured communities there is a propensity for ascribing magic powers to words. Once one enters the field of belief argument is of no avail. The rational thing is to leave the prerogative of using the word "diagnosis" to the medical profession. Speech therapists use their powers of perception to reach a judgement based on scrutiny and appraisal. This process will be called "evaluation". The same dictionary defines "evaluation" as follows: "To ascertain the value or amount of; to appraise carefully".

Logopedists have to appraise carefully, to ascertain the amount of the handicap and loss of value of the individual suffering therefrom. That is evaluation. If by use of this word in preference to diagnosis we can avoid dispute – a war of words about words – good sense and goodwill will have been shown.

Scrutiny and appraisal

Mol (1960) has pointed out that the human organism is less efficient than modern instruments for perception, analysis and reproduction of sound. None the less the human race perforce must use what it has evolved for purposes of communication. Talking cannot be delegated to Universal Robots altogether.

Steer (1960) has given an account of the considerable variety of instruments available for the scrutiny and appraisal of speech. Instruments are indubitably efficient for the purposes of quantitive appraisal and provide a contribution to qualitative criteria. Judgement will for many a long year remain the prerogative of the human race.

Human beings are needed to work apparatus and interpret its information. Complete diagnosis and evaluation require a huge team of experts, with or without costly and complex instruments. The whole team may be required in each case for purposes of research though it is very doubtful that this would be so in each and every case. The patient who seeks treatment must not be subjected to a series of investigations regardless of their relevance unless, exceptionally, he agreed to be a subject for research. For complex and baffling cases it is desirable to have a centre where there is up to date equipment and a team of experts to diagnose the cause of disorders of voice, speech and language, to evaluate the disorders in question and their effect on the sufferer.

Obviously not each and every speech therapy centre can be so equipped and staffed, even in the most affluent society. Diagnostic centres will have to be sited where they can serve a considerable area and large sections of the population. In the United Kingdom a dozen is the largest number we could use. It is quite unlikely that we shall achieve that number. Three or four could prove sufficient. What is wanted most is one for a start.

Such a centre will be costly to build, equip and maintain. The question arises, who will provide it? Will it be the task of the state, as part of our welfare services? Or will state funds be provided indirectly through the universities? Will it be industry that endows it? Or must we hope for private munificence?

Of what value is such a centre to industry? There does not seem to be much likelihood that grants will come from that source. How much capital and annual expenditure will be available from state welfare funds in an era of ever recurring economies in the public sector? Perhaps universities will devote some of their grants to the scheme, but they have many other calls on their resources. Probably we shall have to look to private munificence.

How would such a centre be used?

A procedure for referral to diagnostic centres must be planned. It will probably be through official channels of the Health or Education Services. It is imperative for the logopedist to have access to the centre without complications.

Preliminary evaluation will have to be carried out at speech therapy centres. The outcome of this evaluation will, in a considerable proportion of cases, enable the speech therapist to reach conclusions and take appropriate therapeutic measures. For the remainder, evaluation will provide cases suitable for investigation at the diagnostic centres. It is improbable that elaborate investigations can be completed in one day. It might be a physical possibility for the staff to do so, but it would prove too great a strain on the patients. Children especially need time to adjust to new surroundings; they must be given time to get used to the centre before formal investigations start. Repeated journeys of fifty miles or more would be unpropitious; hence there must be residential facilities for mothers and children there. The speech therapist ought to be present throughout the investigations, but is unlikely to be able to be absent from all other duties for several days. For preference the speech therapist should be present at the preliminary case conference, yet sometimes it may only prove practicable to send a written report in at this stage. It is essential for the speech therapist responsible for the patients to attend the final case conference and hear all the findings; it would be useless at this stage to rely solely on written reports and recommendations.

Anyone referring patients to the centres must be conversant with their equipment and the procedures followed there, even if not expert in the use of the apparatus. The staff at the centre may be mainly or solely interested in the pursuit of knowledge. Those responsible for treatment have to be more pragmatical in their approach. Information of the kind the centre supplies would be useless to anyone not cognisant of its full significance and with no appreciation of the manner in which the findings were reached. On the other hand the staff at the centre would not prescribe definite therapeutic measures, but would recognize that these are the responsibility of the logopedist. Appropriate treatment depends on correct diagnosis; the diagnostician and the practitioner are counterparts: they are not in the position of superior and subordinate.

The existence of centres here envisaged will make ever greater demands on the resourcefulness of speech therapists and on their proficiency, both in devising and applying therapeutic procedures. With effective diagnosis the rationale of treatment must become more clearly defined, less tentative; the treatment itself will not be more routine than it is now.

In the meantime

What is to be done in the meantime? Answer – "Do it yourself". One cannot evade the issue that causes have effects. A variety of causes appear to have similar effects. Careful appraisal facilitates distinction between the similar and the identical. Even without elaborate apparatus, given conditions can be identified and decisions on procedures for their relief reached. In so doing the axiom that the patient, not the symptom, needs treatment must always be borne in mind. One has to use one's eyes and ears, one's hands too, one's knowledge and intelligence with a judicious admixture of insight and intuition. The ear is of supreme importance, since communication by audible signals (and failures thereof), are the logopedist's chief concern. Confronted with a child whose speech development has not followed normal lines, the first thing to do is to listen, and to note the signals he emits, before attending to those he fails to emit.

The phonetic characteristics of the speech of children whose impaired hearing has prevented them from receiving accurately the patterns of sound emitted by others differ from those of children who, though able to receive the signals, fail to apprehend them. In the former, output matches input. The changes of sound pattern are consistent even if varied. In the latter the changes are inconsistent; word-sound patterns vary at random. The failure in output is related to cerebral failure on the input pathways. Comprehension of the verbal symbol exists, but a distorted version of its meaning is derived from it. Where distortion of the signals is due to abnormalities of the executive organs and nervous pathways its characteristics are evident to the sense of hearing of the listener. The eye too has a large part to play and the hand proves useful in examining the organs involved. The characteristics of palatal defects, for example, are easily detected. Dysphonia is another instance of the usefulness of the sense of hearing for the purposes of evaluation. To distinguish, in children, language deviations that are mainly of executive type, investigation by means of the logopedist's senses is likely to be of value. Observation of the manner in which the rhythm of speech is disrupted will as much as anything else help to differentiate cases of cluttering from stammering. To assess the kind of stammering, namely, to differentiate stammering that has evolved on a basis of cluttering (cluttering-stammering) from stammering as a form of learned behaviour or as a psycho-neurotic manifestation, to use one's own senses together with judgement of information acquired from other sources, once more is a sensible procedure. For written language, looking obviously takes the place of listening.

To make an adequate evaluation a great deal of time is needed. If patients are referred with but little useful information, those responsible for referral must be made to admit that full information is needed, that the speech therapists are entitled to the information and must be given the means to obtain it. The attitude "This child cannot speak; teach it" is utterly out of date. It was never justifiable.

REFERENCES

Mol, H. (1960) "De Zwakste Schakel" (The Weakest Link), *Logopedie en Phoniatrie*, Nos. 1, 2 and 3

Steer, M. D. (1960) "Modern Instrumentation for Diagnosis, Therapy and Research", *Folia Phoniatrica* **12**, No. 3 (Paper read at the 11th International Congress of Logopedics and Phoniatrics)

10

C. H. ALDRIDGE, Shrewsbury

Sign-Posts in Diagnosis – Application of the Logoscope

I believe it is true to say that, in the normal course of their work, the majority of speech therapists will not have come across the instrument known as the logoscope.

A form of this instrument is in use as an aid to medical diagnosis. It is described by its inventor, Dr F. A. Nash, as a "panoramic combination index to textbook data", and its aim is to enable a doctor to see, very simply, the differential diagnostic possibilities of the group of signs and symptoms manifested by a patient.

The medical logoscope takes the form of a slide rule. Down one side there is a reference index of disease categories, and by the side of this may be inserted several sign and symptom strips. These strips, which are stored in the back of the instrument, are vertical columns, each labelled with the name of a sign or symptom. Transverse lines on the face of each strip indicate, when it is in place on the front of the instrument, those diseases in which that particular manifestation has been described. That is, the lines are marked on each column at the level of those diseases. When several strips are inserted together some of these lines will coincide, forming a horizontal line across some or all of the strips, showing that all of those signs and symptoms have been described in the disease adjacent to that line.

Thus, the doctor, having selected and inserted the strips for the symptoms of which his patient is complaining and the signs which he is presenting, is able to see immediately the differential diagnostic possibilities and probabilities of the case. A study of these will indicate certain lines of inquiry to be followed in the history taking, and probably further investigations to be undertaken.

Dr Nash gives the following example of the way in which the logoscope helps the physician:

A patient complains of colicky pain, headache and recent constipation. He also reports that his gums bleed at times. The doctor's examination suggests anaemia, and there is a slow pulse. To make use of the logoscope, the strips for these manifestations are selected and inserted into the face of the instrument. There are many lines on each strip showing the diseases in which occur the symptoms that have been described. In fact, there are over four hundred lines on these six strips, but the doctor will find that a horizontal line is formed by all six at one place only. The condition adjacent to that line is plumbism. Armed with this clue, the doctor will then question the patient further, to establish his connection with any form of lead, and will be able to confirm this diagnosis by tests to estimate the lead content of the patient's urine.

Document-copying equipment may be used to produce a record of the pattern shown on the logoscope. This record is called a logogram, and can be filed with the patient's case-notes. Logograms made at intervals during the course of a disease provide a useful check on the progress being made, and any changes of data which may occur.

It is obvious that this instrument is not needed for every patient, but rather where immediate recognition of the condition does not take place. Neither is it intended to furnish a complete diagnosis, but to narrow down the field. As Dr Nash explains, it can be described metaphorically as a diagnostic bus and not a diagnostic taxi, in that the user will find that it often takes him near to his diagnostic destination but not, usually, from door to door. He also stresses that it is not a substitute for textbooks and clinical knowledge. On the contrary, a good physician will make better use of the logoscope than a poor one. The logoscope takes the place of time-consuming sifting through textbooks. It does not eliminate the necessity to recall one's experience of similar cases, or descriptions read of cases which have something in common with the one under examination. Dr Nash points out that "more is missed through not recalling, and so not looking, than through not knowing".

The logoscope, therefore, provides a very valuable sign-post along the diagnostic way for the physician since it has a knowledge of the prima differentia. Could it also point the way for the speech therapist?

This question was posed by a research group of Midland speech therapists, and they decided that it would make an interesting subject for investigation. They were all fully occupied with other projects for this Conference however, and very generously invited me to explore the possibilities of a logoscope as an aid to the diagnosis of speech disorders.

It was thought that only one speech disorder should be considered in this investigation into the application of logoscopy to our work. In this pilot inquiry the choice was stammering, and it was decided to follow Dr Nash's method of collecting data. That is, that the manifestations of stammering should be listed, as well as the other conditions in which some of these manifestations appear. Thus, for the logoscope, each manifestation would be written on a separate strip, and the conditions would be listed down the side.

First of all then, the manifestations of the sign-symptom complex referred to as stammering.

Much has has been written and much has been argued about the causes and treatment of this condition. Less has been said, however, about the symptoms themselves. Few textbooks give comprehensive details. Any reader who had never come across stammering would find it difficult to get a really good picture from some of the available literature.

Admittedly, faced with the problem of describing stammering to someone who had never heard of it, most of us would find it easier to imitate some of the symptoms, than to describe them in words. Descriptions of stammering tend to become confused with explanations.

In those books where more detailed accounts are given, the tendency is to do so only in connection with specific patients, and the signs and symptoms described do not therefore lead to a *general* description, i.e. to the construction of a model of the disorder.

It may be that many people agree with Franklin Brook who says, "There are many observations one can make relative to the behaviour of the typical stammerer. They do not help us to plan any effective treatment however." Those of us who have not had the advantage of Brook's experience with stammerers, and believing that treatment is likely to be effective only if applied to the right patient, may feel that more observations would help us to be confident that we are, in fact, dealing with an idiopathic stammer. The scarcity of specific details of the symptoms of stammering may be due to the fact that there are so many variations of this condition. Writers may feel that if they attempted to describe every type of stammer there would be no room in their books for anything else! Certainly, one point on which everyone will agree is that no two stammerers are alike.

At first glance, this would seem to be a contra-indication for the use of a logoscope. Further examination of this point, however, indicates that the value of applying logoscopy to the study of stammering lies in this very fact. What is needed for the logoscope is a list of the possible manifestations of stammering, not a list of the different types of stammer. The category reference index of the logoscope will provide a list of diseases and disorders in which one or more of the manifestations that comprise the "stammer complex" have been described. Dr Nash explains that every medical case is in many ways unique, since individual aspects will be unclassifiable, and no patient will have *all* the symptoms of a disease described in the textbooks. All the aspects of stammering cannot be unique by virtue of the fact that they are classified as stammer symptoms.

The following list of manifestations is submitted as a possible one from which sign and symptom strips could be made. An attempt has been made to group them as far as possible, since this would make them easier to find in practice.

Signs manifested by stammerers

CONCERNING VOICE:
Sudden variations in pitch
High-pitched voice
Low-pitched voice
Variations in intensity
Loud voice
Very quiet voice, or whispering
Use of monotone

CONCERNING RESPIRATION:
  Irregular respiratory pattern during speech
  Speech on residual breath
  Speech on inspiration
  Breath held

REPETITIONS:
  1. Uncontrolled: rhythmical repetition of sounds in the word being spoken
  Rhythmical repetition of syllables of words being spoken
  Rhythmical repetition of noises made with tongue, or lips, or velum (i.e. other than accepted speech sounds – "clicks")
  2. Deliberate: repetition of previous word, or phrase, or sentence

HESITATIONS:
  Delayed initiation of speech
  Slight pauses between words
  Pause with glottal stop
  Pause with vocalization
  Prolongation of sounds in the words being spoken
  Pause with the use of an "easy" word e.g. "well". Pause with the use of coughs, "ums", "ers", etc.

RATES OF SPEECH:
  Slow and deliberate
  Very rapid

ARTICULATION:
  Precise – paying too much attention to sound production
  Forceful
  Slurred
  Omission of certain sounds

EXCESSIVE MUSCULAR MOVEMENTS:
  1. Uncontrolled, during speech. (Spasms) of: tongue, lips, jaw, eyes, facial muscles, throat muscles, head, shoulders, arms, hands, trunk, muscles of respiration, legs, feet
  2. Deliberate, during speech. (Assisting mechanisms) of: tongue, lips, jaw, eyes, facial muscles, throat muscles, head, shoulders, arms, hands, trunk, muscles of respiration, legs, feet
  3. Tremors of: hands, lips, tongue
  4. Tics

SYNTAX:
- Order of words changed
- Sentences condensed – telegrammic

REACTION TO SPEECH PROBLEM:
- Embarrassed
- Struggles to overcome difficulty
- Sometimes gives up completely

EMOTIONAL:
- Failure to look at listener
- Blushing
- Sweating
- Self-consciousness
- Nervousness
- Anxious
- Suspicious
- Tense

Symptoms reported by stammerers

Inability to: Get words out, say certain words, say certain sounds, speak to certain people, speak in certain situations
Difficulty with reading
Difficulty with spelling
Evades words which he fears he will be unable to say – substitutes others
Speech worse when tired
Has premonitions of stammer
Experiences sensations in parts of speech musculature during stammering
Experiences visceral sensations
Worries about speech
Avoids speech situations
Is irritable

It is not suggested that this is anything but a tentative list. No doubt many modifications and additions would be necessary before a final one could be agreed upon. In its preparation, considerable difficulty was experienced in finding satisfactory words to describe the manifestations. Adaptation of neurological terms is popular with some therapists, but this is not at all suitable for the purpose of logoscopy. The attempt to utilize this system of organizing data indicates the need for a truly scientific terminology.

Van Riper mentions a German authority which described ninety-two different varieties of stammering, and he adds that there must be many more. The manifestations listed here would produce more than a hundred million different combinations!

It now becomes clear that logoscopy is of great potential value in the field of stammering quite apart from its importance in differential diagnosis. The use of logograms would enable us to record, very simply, most of the aspects of a patient's stammer, to note any changes which may occur, to compare different patterns of stammering and to classify them according to their structure rather than their descriptive features.

Returning to diagnosis, attention must now be given to the other conditions in which these manifestations are found. It was interesting to discover that, with the exception of alalia and severe forms of aphasia, this list includes all other speech conditions. It is thought that, as a guide to therapists investigating cases of stammering, it would be useful to include certain psychiatric conditions, such as paranoia, anxiety neurosis and hysteria. A predominance of features of any of these conditions would indicate to the therapist that a psychiatrist's opinion should be sought before any speech therapy is attempted, just as a predominance of the features of Parkinsonian dysarthria would prompt her to refer the case to a neurologist.

It may be thought that an experienced speech therapist is well able to recognize a stammer without the aid of a logoscope. The numbers of unsuccessfully treated cases, however, may be an indication of some errors in diagnosis. It is as well to bear in mind that Russian therapists, writing in *Speech* in 1937, stated that the number of cases sent to them diagnosed as stammering and found to be organic lesions of the central nervous system was very large. The differential diagnostic possibilities of stammering symptoms are well worth consideration and, again, may lead to new developments in research.

The advantages of applying the system of logoscopy to the study of stammering have been pointed out. In many aspects of speech and language new developments are taking place, and the number of differential diagnostic possibilities is increasing rapidly. More speech therapists are placing greater emphasis on initial investigation and for them a logoscope would be a great asset in that it would provide a systematic method of investigation, save treatment time, and probably save the patient's time. It would also mean that, in certain cases, a patient would not be discouraged by lack of progress due to the wrong method of treatment. These are some of the obvious advantages and more will undoubtedly be revealed by further study of the full application of logoscopy in the field of speech disorders.

Could the logoscope also point the way for the speech therapist? This preliminary investigation indicates that the answer will be "Yes".

I wish to thank Dr Nash for his interest and assistance in this project and my colleagues who gave me the opportunity to undertake it. I am particularly grateful to Dr Stein, who first brought the logoscope to the attention of the Research Group.

REFERENCES

Brook, Franklin (1958) *Stammering and its Treatment*, London, Pitman Medical

Florenskaya, Y. A., Averbukh, I. S., and Arkhipoua, O. G. (1937) "Some Difficult Cases of Stammering", *Speech* **3**, No. 1

Nash, F. A. (1954) "Differential Diagnosis", *Lancet*, April 24

Nash, F. A. (1959) "Talking Sense", *Lancet*, Oct. 17.

Nash, F. A. (1960) "Diagnostic Reasoning", *Lancet*, Dec. 31

11

PEGGY CARTER, London

The Suppression of the Signal

The suppression of the signal refers here to stammering. As I see it, the tension involved in a stammer indicates the suppression of a signal which, coming from the unconscious, would betray, were it unsuppressed, a state of mind which would acutely embarrass the speaker.

Let us first inquire what is meant by a signal. It is an allusive act or behaviour which is an indication or warning of something else. A stammer involves deliberate or conscious acts designed to prevent the manifestation of an unconscious state of the psyche of which the stammerer is, or would be, deeply ashamed if it were signalled or alluded to.

Stammering can hardly be regarded or even described as a speech defect.

It certainly is not a constant one which lends itself to speech correction exercises. One has never met a stammerer who could not speak fluently in certain circumstances. In so far as it is one, it is concerned with an extra-verbal aspect of speech.

What we say is not only a verbalization of our thoughts. The kinds of things we say and the way we say them are governed in large part by our relationship with the person we are with, our relative position, intellect, general status and so on, and on our right to make demands and to speak freely.

Experience has shown me that the stammerer has to a large extent remained in a state of infantile omnipotence. If we scratch his outer covering, which may be one of humility, we find the arrogance and demanding character belonging to an infant in arms who demands to be waited upon better than any king and is sadly irked by having to give way to anyone.

Omnipotence means "all powerfulness" but the stammerer is totally unaware, that is, unconscious, of the infantile nature of his demand for power. It is, however, betrayed in such remarks as "If I could speak I should reach the stars", "If I could speak everything would be all right," "If I could speak I should be able to earn big money and make my parents happy." These and many other remarks are frequently made.

I therefore contend that the signal suppressed by the stammerer points to his right to absolute power in the social situation; it expresses that the speaker, feeling and believing this fantasy power, is humiliated and frightened when he is opposed by power with a basis of reality. It is then that the signal which says, more or less, "I am the king of the castle, get down you dirty rascal" is suppressed so that the fearful incongruity of his demands shall not be realized by those to whom he is speaking, and certainly not by the speaker himself.

Incongruity, according to Herbert Spencer, is the basis for laughter. We must realize that the stammerer's sensitiveness to it is more highly charged than is warranted by laughter at the defect itself. When the stammerer has confidence in the therapist and can express himself freely, the incongruity is seen between the stammerer's infantile demand for recognition of his importance and the real situation. In view of the absurdity of his attitude, the stammerer does very well to suppress it.

The signal conveys a claim for power for the stammerer on easy terms. It also conveys the repudiation of power in others. This repudiation of other people's rights to power would of course be most deeply felt in the stammerer's relations to any "V.I.P." including the boss, and to others in a superior position. Such claims for power are satisfied most fully by the mother with her child at the breast.

No doubt the power problem is common to the whole human race and it is difficult to draw a line between the man in the street and these problematical patients of ours, but observations carried out over a number of years have shown that in stammerers it is greatly accentuated. I have acted on this realization in treatment and believe my assumption regarding the powerful factor at work to be true. Since I feel that the stammerer's character problem is typified by his attitude to power, let us look at its distribution and the attitude to it in his home where he has formed his early impressions, to see if we can find a common characteristic there. I believe we can.

In this regard the most typical and outstanding fact is that the mother herself does not accept the male dominance of her husband. More often than not the stammerer cooperates in this state of affairs, perhaps too much so. At times a fair adjustment is made but sometimes the sparks fly; the mother may retreat into negativity or the father may be dead or absent (although these last two factors constitute an altogether different problem). Quite commonly the mother achieves her position by kindness, general force of character or by competence or ability greater than that of her husband, but in any case the power of the husband is rejected and the mother generally exhibits an over-supply of what the Jungian theory calls "animus".

How does this affect the child? Perhaps in two ways. First, his own power drive is not supported by the father pattern which he sees at home. Secondly his mother has made her choice of a mate by whom she will not be dominated. How then will she stand being dominated by her own child? Will he not deduce from the way she handles him that his only power is the power of helplessness, and, according to his character, fight against it or submit to it?

Let us consider the first point first, if only because the father's attitude in the family reflects the child at a later age and is more available to consciousness; we may therefore more easily assess its influence and can approach it more openly in treatment.

The male patient can often see that he has not been able to assume his full masculine role and exercise his full power because he has not had at home a father pattern on which he can model himself. His realization of the reasons for his angry repudiation of the father often helps to lower the patient's feeling of guilt. The girl, on the other hand, may have modelled herself too well on the mother and she finds not only that her mother objects but that her assumption of the right to dominate is not welcome to associates and seniors. The power signals in her case, too, must be suppressed to avoid ridicule.

The second point takes us back to the root of the matter. The mother, I postulate, does not fancy domination and this has influenced her choice of a partner; nor will she fancy being dominated by the will of her child. Neither the child's own will to power nor that of his father is acceptable to the love object, his mother. Therefore it receives no sanction of any kind and is subjected to repression.

This problem is certainly far more difficult than the previous one to approach in treatment. Stammering is an oral symptom, and the power of the child over his mother is expressed on the oral plane from his earliest days. The influence is felt at the breast before the dawn of a consciousness ordinarily available to memory. To be effective in bringing about a symptom, however, the experience will have to be reinforced in a number of ways throughout his formative life; the symptom indeed may only be touched off by some threat to self-regard in much later days. The repressed unconscious, however, remains dynamic within the psyche, and the repressed idea returns as a symptom expressing that the stammerer seeks oral power throughout his life.

The child's repudiation of his father as a power figure seems to be common to all stammerers but sometimes this seems to be contradicted by a very much loved father. On close inquiry, however, we usually find that the father is playing the part of a second mother or nanny, which is very usual in the child's earliest infancy, especially in these days of no servants. The real task of the father is, however, to bring his children face to face with reality. He often plays the part of second mother very charmingly, for the man who is good with children is, on the whole, an attractive character, and may very likely be supplying the warmth that he feels is lacking in his wife. The child's repudiation of the father has a notable exception in the case of the father who is dead or absent, but the situation is different, for the father remains a fantasy. He is endowed in the child's imagination with plenty of power but it is to subdue the wife and not the child itself. The child remains without the tempering fire of having to submit to the father's acknowledged strength through which he, the child, graduates to a realization of his own strength. It is this tempering fire which teaches a child to develop his strength (physical or mental), and to achieve power without expecting it the easy way on infantile terms.

There are events in the child's life which may trigger off or accentuate a stammer. One of these is entry into school, thus coming face to face with new hierarchies. Certainly among the touching-off points I number learning to read, for in reading aloud speech has to share its oral quality with a visual one and must follow a discipline governed by an arrangement of a row of letters. The child, especially the orally fixated one, feels that in the act of speech he has great power. Reading aloud is a threat to the freedom of his oral satisfaction which is often deeply resented; sometimes the task of learning to read is even rejected so that he cannot learn to read or to develop the kind of vocabulary learned through literature. In my view this is the explanation of the poor verbal ability said to be found among these patients, rather than the presence of any neurological anomaly.

On reaching the junior school and leaving behind the far freer and more talkative infant classes the stammerer's orality is once more threatened. (How often, to our surprise, is the stammerer in trouble for talking in class, the last thing we would expect from someone with a stultifying speech defect about which he is so grossly sensitive.) He may also see applied to others, and thus may expect for himself, aggression in the form of corporal punishment. Aggression begets aggression and he feels his own infantile omnipotent feelings stirring once more, only to be met once again with the sensation of powerlessness so deeply accepted whenever it is experienced.

In conclusion some cases may be quoted to illustrate the points made. The statement that all stammerers can speak fluently under certain conditions appeared to be contradicted by a patient who for a whole year asserted that in his case it was certainly not true. This patient assured me that his stammer was always the same whether he was talking to himself, the dog, his family, his boss, indeed everyone. One day he came crestfallen and reported that a dictaphone had been introduced into the office; on playing back his dictation he found that his speech had been perfect until somebody came into the room when he immediately began to stammer. Significantly, he left me after this episode. He had triumphantly killed off at least seven speech therapists and had one of the most watertight stammers and stammering attitudes I had ever come across. It was obvious from the first that he had no intention of ever attempting to get rid of his stammer. There was absolute resistance here to the power of the mother (and thus of his woman therapist). His mother and his elder sister had been extremely powerful in his young life when his father was in the war-time Navy. The father in this case was an interesting figure; he sent home books from the other side of the world full of illustrated stories which he wrote and drew for his children. He was a very warm and loving man but one who expressed mainly his womanly side. For instance, at the time of the patient's treatment he spent most of his leisure time on the womanly art of weaving. I had the impression that the patient's great desire in childhood had been for his father to come home and assert his masculine power and liberate the power of the patient so that together they might fight the mother's power. This never happened. The mother was beautiful, the father loved her and conceived his love as one that should always give way. The family appeared to be an ideal one. Out of love for his father, it seems, my patient clamped down on his rebellion and clamped his speech down with it. But his will to power over his speech therapist even in a negative sense was quite exceptionally evident – a very strong transference from the mother.

However, I treated him incorrectly. He had far more fantasy than most stammerers and I should have allowed him to give vent to fantasy rather than treat him through interpretation and discussion. After the first resistance there was some easing in the relationship, some tendency to confide, but the slightest comment on my part would close the door on that particular confidence and the door could not be reopened. He feared my intrusion and I should have played a passive role. However, to do this is so seldom effective with stammerers, who usually need the therapist to play an active part nearer to their active mother (at least at first), that I did not realize it in time and I lost my chance. He was a delightful creature who may well be one of the few stammerers who would know what to do with an anima figure if he met one.

The signal probably was "I must induce mother to become a woman". This was bitten hard back but with rather less fear of ridicule than with most stammerers. He got on well with his fellow men, he was not bullied and would never have appeared a figure of fun. He could not, however, achieve his task without his father's help and sanction.

Here is another case with a fantasy father who was killed at Dunkirk when the children were three. (My patient had a twin sister.) To this patient his father was an idealized figure; he dreamed, for instance, of a golden coloured Churchill sitting in the House of Commons. His father had indeed been successful, a public school and University rowing man, a yachtsman, a member of Lloyds, a social king and one who carried all before him. My patient did not compete. He became an artist and used to come to his treatment up to the forehead in paint and none too clean. He was, in fact, Bohemian in dress, thoroughly different from his polished father. Here are three of his dreams. The final one before treatment ceased is given first. He was one of three men going to take their places in a modern streamlined transparent boat. There was no doubt about the place for one of them, an insignificant school fellow, who took that of the lightest man in the bows. The other man, however, was an artist and friend who had figured considerably in our discussions in the early days of treatment as a natural leader of men. In this dream there was some doubt as to which of them should row stroke, the man who sets the rhythm (let us realize how important this question of rhythm is, as well as the dominating position of stroke!) and which of them should be second, which is the place of the strongest rower. In the end my patient took the place of second and strongest, but he would have been able to take the other place. Dreaming of boats had always referred to his father (the rowing man and yachtsman) and the streamlined modern boat seemed to mean that he had brought the power conflict into his own generation and out of the past; the transparency signified that he had insight.

In his penultimate dream, a long one and full of significance, but too complicated to go into in full, my patient dreamed that the woman friend who could give him the introduction to leading artists (power figures) in Cornwall, where he was going to live, had her baby with her and was feeding it, but very clumsily and doing it all wrong. He thought perhaps the baby was too slow.

The same patient had another dream some months earlier (treatment was always intermittent after the initial period, since he had long Slade holidays in Cornwall as well as other interruptions). He and his wife had bought a house in Cornwall and in the dream this house, instead of being on the mainland, was on the Scilly Isles which were not, as they are in reality, out of sight of land but could be seen with great clarity with only a very narrow channel of water between them and the mainland. He was waiting with his mother to take her over by the usual steamer to see the new house when he suddenly realized that he could go over by a coal barge which would be much nicer. But his mother would not go on anything so dirty. Islands often symbolize the ego, and certainly the patient had this dream at a time when his ego was beginning to emerge.

This patient had always been out of sympathy with his conventional mother who had, it seemed, been more natural with the twin sister than with him. His guilt was about slowness at the breast. Perhaps he needed to linger there and keep his mother longer from his twin. The signal he wished to make was for us all to await his leisured pace at the breast, showing his desire to linger there. For this to be acted out he also needed his mother to appreciate him in the childish stage where dirt, carelessness and messing about are accepted. This is exactly the stage he was caught in when he realized that he must compete with the golden figure of his father's ghost for his mother's love.

Another case is of a young girl of nineteen with a stammer and dysarthria, smart and pretty as a picture, with a cerebellar defect, spasticity and a severe hearing loss. Her daydream, of which she could not have been more ashamed, was to be employed as a nude in a Paris revue. It is to be noted that she wanted to achieve power through her one priceless asset, a beautiful body. No men fell for this crippled girl and she could not talk with them, but she knew she could win love for her body and signalled by her stammer "come and get me". Although she could not have stood still on her legs for two minutes and, with her upbringing, would have run crying from the scene in terror if faced with the reality, this did not interfere with her daydream. Unfortunately she is now also losing her sight and the diagnosis is that of hereditary familial ataxia. Significantly enough with the loss of sight she has also lost her stammer. Although the dysarthria is organic, no doubt remains regarding the psychological nature of her stammer. The signal is no longer necessary now that the pathetic power of the blind, the power of helplessness, is hers.

12

M. J. L. ELLIS, London

Breakdown in Communication in a Nine-Year-Old Boy

The modern science of language defines linguistic communication as a system of signals, signs and symbols by which people have agreed to abide. In order to understand any breakdown of this system it is necessary to define it also in terms of its evolution and development.

The higher animals other than man also possess a means of communicating with each other but the content of such communication is strictly limited to the transfer from one to another of the feeling tone of the moment, that is, the sounds the animal emits, or its bodily postures, are signals of its emotional state; such signals may be interpreted as signs of certain things by those who know the animal well but the capacity of the animal to use signs is actually very limited and animals are incapable of producing symbols.

The human infant is equipped with an innate capacity to emit signals. Lip smacking, expressing pleasure, is present from the earliest weeks, and so are cries whose volume, pitch and timbre vary according to whether they express rage, pain or frustration. Such noises are signals expressive of the infant's emotional state and are not intentional; to the experienced mother who can interpret them, however, they may well come as signs asking her to do something. In the course of his language development the child learns to emit verbal signs intentionally and as his communication becomes purposive, the expression of his emotional state through signals ebbs. Nonetheless, as may be expected from its long phylogenetic ancestry, the form of expression depicting feeling is very deeply rooted in the nervous system and is never entirely lost from human speech – witness the involuntary "oo" of pain and the range of vocal inflection in adult speech.

Hughlings Jackson (1958) describes evolution as the passage from the most to the least organized, from the most fossilized to the most flexible, from the most consolidated to the least consolidated, from the most simple to the most complex, from the most automatic to the most voluntary. Dissolution, a term introduced by him into medicine, Jackson defined as being the reverse of the process of evolution – a process of undevelopment, a breaking down in order from the least organized, from the most complex and most voluntary towards the most organized, most simple and most automatic. Jackson considered that unless dissolution is total, resulting in death, some level of evolution is left though not necessarily in its original form.

Stein (1953), who applied Jackson's doctrine to speech and language, postulated that if the top levels of language ceased for any reason to function normally, the action patterns of the well-canalized lower levels would be released. I should like now to examine, from the standpoint of these theories, the case of a nine-year-old boy.

Gavin A., an intelligent only child, was nine years eight months old when he was referred to the clinic. Sometimes his speech was normal and fluent, but it was held up at other times by a prolonged glottal stop. While this lasted, the boy would cease whatever he was doing, his facial expression would be one of acute terror with mouth and eyes wide open. When he was unoccupied or reading to himself, Gavin would suck the lapel of his jacket noisily; if asked not to do so, he would desist but start to produce sharp lip-smacking noises. A third symptom consisted in tuneless humming interjected by noisy swallowing.

Gavin was a pale, stiff, spotlessly clean boy with a precise, unchildlike manner – a favourite remark of his, made in a pompous tone, was "Of course, so-and-so is too young for me". This usually referred to some activity that should have been quite normal at his age. Unlike many boys, he used restraint in his choice of words and was careful never to make a sweeping statement. He replied politely to my remarks to him but made few on his own initiative and was obviously embarrassed by our conversation. He gave the impression of mentally edging away. This inability to let himself go and to make a warm feeling contact with another person was not confined to the speech therapy clinic; Gavin was described by his parents as silent, very reserved and unable to show his feelings. In situations where he might be expected to show pleasure, affection or anger he registered nothing. He was habitually stiff and uneasy with adults, reluctant to make contacts with other boys and never played freely. He would not go to the shops or cinema alone and usually waited until one of his parents could accompany him. A report from Gavin's school confirmed this picture but added that Gavin's behaviour was satisfactory and his school work good.

The parents were a well-balanced, affectionate couple and the root of Gavin's difficulties appeared to lie in the past circumstances of the family's life rather than in their present handling of him. Gavin had been a sickly, anaemic baby who had cried an excessive amount until he was eighteen months old. From his birth until he was four years of age, the housing shortage had forced the family to live with Gavin's maternal grandparents and because his cries disturbed her mother, Mrs. A. had tried constantly to quieten not only these but also any other loud noise the boy made. She had finally succeeded and the noisy baby had grown into an over-quiet toddler who was late in starting to speak. When Gavin was four years old, he and his parents went to live with his aged great-grandparents. This couple, who were over eighty, couldn't stand noise and Mrs A. once more felt obliged to say "hush" and "don't" to Gavin. Because there were no neighbouring children with whom he could play, and because his great-grandparents' frailty made it impossible to invite children to the house, Gavin led not only a silent but also an abnormally secluded existence.

Thus the normal outlets of aggressiveness and emotion had been taboo to Gavin almost since birth. Small wonder that he was unable to express his feelings or to relate normally to other people. Matters had improved to some extent by the time I saw the boy since the paternal grandparents had died one year previously and Gavin and his parents had then, for the first time, acquired their own home. The effect of his early experiences was, however, so deeply ingrained that the change of environment had brought about only a partial improvement in Gavin's personality.

Where does the speech disturbance fit into this picture? This had started when Gavin was five years four months old. At that time he was admitted to the Infant School and, unprepared for this by any previous contact with other children or experience of life outside his home, he found it terrifying. The other children, sensing no doubt that Gavin was "different", did not accept him and he met with much unkindness from them. One day, a group of children set upon him on the way home from school. Unused to standing up for himself, Gavin apparently made no attempt to defend himself and was found later by his mother who had come to look for him, crouching in the gutter, more shaken than actually hurt. The glottal stop was heard for the first time by Mrs A. when Gavin tried to tell her what had occurred. The sucking, lip smacking and swallowing noises began shortly afterwards.

To understand the meaning of Gavin's symptoms, we must consider first one of the basic functions of the larynx. Negus (1929) has pointed out that it is incorrect and misleading to speak of the larynx as an organ of voice since it is primarily a valve which by firm closure during the act of swallowing prevents the possible intrusion of foreign bodies such as food and water into the lower respiratory tract. This function of the larynx, common only to man, whose larynx and oesophagus are at the same anatomical level, is as old as mankind – that is, roughly one million years old. The closure of the larynx is therefore a very deeply canalized pattern, seen in human beings in response to sudden fright. Stein (1949, 1951) has shown that the glottal stop, a by-product of the closure of the larynx as a protection against the intrusion of foreign bodies, may be used to keep out symbolically something that cannot be dealt with in reality; it is therefore a classic anxiety symptom.

Such appeared to be the meaning of Gavin's glottal stop. He was afraid of people and of venturing into the world and unable even to express his fears. Because he could not cope with life in reality he produced the glottal stop as a symbolical means of keeping out the intruders that he feared. It also served to keep in the hostility and aggression that he feared to express and, indeed, did not even recognize in himself. It is not surprising that the glottal stop should be produced shortly after he had had to face an apparently hostile, dangerous outside world for the first time and immediately after the most terrifying experience in his life. It was noticeable at the time I knew him that experiences he particularly feared, for instance, a visit to the dentist, were always met with apparent stoicism and a markedly high frequency of the glottal stop. The involuntary expression of terror that accompanied the hold up underlined the fact that it was related to a feeling of fear.

Lip smacking and sucking noises are linguistic signals expressive of the most rudimentary feeling relationship – that of the infant with his mother. From these infantile sounds some consonant sounds gradually grow as Stein (1949, 1951) has shown. Noisy swallowing also belongs to this level. It seemed that, as a result of his early experiences, Gavin's feeling was still infantile. Unable to form the relationships appropriate to his years, his feeling was expressed instead in these very primitive signals. Under the stress of emotional disturbance, normal verbal communication had broken down and, in conformity with the doctrines of Jackson and Stein, dissolution or regression to the fossilized primitive level of signals had taken place.

Neither Gavin nor those around him, of course, attributed this meaning to his signals. Both he and his parents regarded his glottal stop as something that prevented him "getting his words out", and his mother often enjoined him in regard to his tics "not to make those noises". Once I knew his history, however, I understood the fear and desire to relate to other people which the signals conveyed. Thus to *me* those signals were signs and my ability to interpret them was a guide to applying an appropriate form of treatment.

In a case such as this, it is obviously useless to work directly upon speech or through relaxation, nor was Gavin old enough for his problem to be tackled through discussion. Play is the natural medium through which children express their ideas and feelings and I therefore decided to see Gavin regularly and to encourage him simply to play in the hope that this would help him to become more child-like and non-verbally expressive. This form of treatment met with no favour from Gavin who protested that he was too old to play. He was reluctant to attend the clinic and persistently forgot, that is, repressed appointments or kept them late. While with me, his eye was on the clock and he never failed to remind me when it was time for him to leave the clinic.

Once I had introduced Gavin to the toys, I did not urge him to use them; I simply took the attitude that it is natural for children to wish to play and awaited developments. Surprisingly soon, Gavin walked over to the sand tray and began very stiffly and self-consciously, to make roads in the sand. This he did for several visits though he would tell me nothing about the roads and seemed half ashamed to be making them. One day, a new element appeared – a gate at the side of the road behind which was a farmyard. Gavin described this gate as "blocked up" and showed concern that it should be so; the farmyard contained animals.

This piece of play was illustrative of Gavin's psychological position. The closed gate was the equivalent of the closure of the larynx; it stopped anyone from getting in and also prevented the egress of the animals, that is, Gavin's natural instinctual side. In response to a suggestion from me, Gavin removed the gate and the effect was almost magical. Not only did the animals pass freely in and out of the farmyard, but Gavin's play changed and became much less inhibited – cars fell into booby traps, planes fought and crashed, cowboys and Indians killed one another. The opening of the gate had evidently freed much previously repressed hostility and aggression.

Although until this point in treatment Gavin had tolerated my presence and had replied to my questions about his play, his attitude had been unmistakably "stand-offish". The release of aggression and hostility appeared now to free in him the ability, hitherto lacking, to show positive feeling towards another person, since, for the first time, he began to take the initiative in making a relationship with me. He began, for instance, to be most anxious for me to notice his play and this was accompanied by a running commentary interspersed by "Look, look, Miss Ellis, watch – are you watching me?" Now, far from forgetting appointments, he arrived early to keep them and could be persuaded only with difficulty to leave when time was up.

As I have already pointed out, Gavin's glottal stop signified, "Keep out, I'm afraid of you". Now of his own free will he was using language to say in effect, "Come in, I want to make friends with you". As this attitude also extended outside the clinic to other adults and children, it is not surprising that Gavin's need to signal decreased and that there was a reduction in frequency of both glottal stop and sucking noises.

Until this point in treatment, Gavin had played only with dry sand; he had ignored the water provided. Now he began cautiously to use it, showing concern when it slopped upon himself or on the floor. When I pointed out to him that he seemed to find it difficult really to "let himself go", he began to use it more freely until about five weeks after he had first introduced it, he was playing in a trough brimming with water. Now began a series of sea games – there were storms at sea, sluice gates opened and let the waters out while water was poured and slopped unrestrainedly. As this freedom developed in his play, Gavin became less and less inhibited in himself. He was increasingly able to express his feelings not only to me but also to his parents and teachers. His caution ebbed and he began to describe people and events in colourful colloquial terms. As he became more and more able to make relationships with other people, so his fear of them and of life outside his home decreased. He began to make friends with other boys, to use public transport and to enter shops alone. As he became increasingly able to accept life and other people and to form normal relationships, his need for the glottal stop, sucking noises, humming and swallowing decreased in frequency and severity and finally disappeared.

Eight months after treatment had started, it was stopped for four months to see how Gavin would get on without regular treatment. Communication was still normal at the end of this time and Gavin was discharged from the speech therapy clinic. Seventeen months later, when he was twelve years three months, his case was followed up and speech was found to be still normal. Gavin was confident, easy in manner and ready to converse. His parents reported a slight temporary set-back upon his entering the Technical School at eleven years four months but otherwise no relapse.

Summary and conclusion

The term "stammer" is not in itself sufficient to clarify the nature of the condition thus designated. In order to explain more fully the nature and meaning of stammer in a nine-year-old boy, use was made of Jackson's doctrine of dissolution, Stein's theory arising from this and also the psychodynamic point of view. It was concluded that under the stress of emotional disturbance, the boy's top levels of communication had broken down and that regression to the primitive level of signalling had taken place. Because the speech therapist was able to interpret the signals produced they were to her signs of certain psychological attitudes. Since his situation could not be discussed with so young a boy, he was treated by play. Play may be described as an organized system of non-verbal symbols and through its medium the boy worked out his psychological problem symbolically. As his attitude became more normal, the boy's need to signal his difficulties decreased and the stammer and allied symptoms abated in frequency and finally disappeared.

REFERENCES

Fordham, Michael (1947) *The Life of Childhood*, London, Kegan Paul

Howe, G. (1931) "Motives and Mechanisms of the Mind", *Lancet*

Jackson, J. H. (1958) *Selected Writings*, London, Staples Press

Negus, V. E. (1929) *The Mechanism of the Larynx*, London, William Heinemann

Orton, S. T. (1937) *Reading, Writing and Speech Disorders in Childhood*, London

Stein, L. (1949) *The Infancy of Speech and the Speech of Infancy*, London, Methuen

Stein, L. (1953) "Stammering as a Psychosomatic Disorder", *Folia Phoniatrica* **5**, No. 1

Stein, L. (1951) "On Talking or the Communication of Ideas and Feelings by means of mainly Audible Symbols", *The British Journal of Medical Psychology* **XXIV**, Part 2

Valentine, C. W. (1942) *The Psychology of Early Childhood*, London, Methuen

13

JOAN POLLITT, Maidstone

Children's drawings, their value in therapy

All well-equipped speech therapy clinics at which children attend have play material – sand, water, toys, crayons and so on. How can this material be used in the child's best interests? I have often heard speech therapists say that when using such material children become at ease, that they look forward to their visits and are happy while in the clinic – that children are stimulated by such material. Obviously no one would despise these effects. Can this material be used for purposes other than the provision of a happy atmosphere? Can the use of such material be the means of relieving a speech disorder?

A therapist who uses drawing and painting or play as a medium through which a change in the speech situation is to be achieved, must first exclude all possibility that either organic abnormality, mental retardation or both is at the root of the speech problem. A drawing-painting play approach to treatment is nevertheless likely to produce some insight and initiative in most children, but such treatment is not likely, of itself, to improve a speech disorder of organic origin or one associated with mental retardation.

In cases where the speech defect is not a symptom of mental retardation and where no organic cause can be diagnosed to account for the speech abnormality, it is reasonable to assume that the disorder is psychological in origin. This can all the more confidently be assumed where, in addition to the speech problem, the child shows symptoms which are readily recognized by parents, teachers and therapists alike as being indicative of psychological maladjustment – for example, symptoms such as timidity, fear of the dark, fear of leaving mother, general lack of confidence and so on.

Experience has taught me that, even if none of these unhappy symptoms exist and even if the home and school environments seem ideal according to conventional standards, a child may still be psychologically maladjusted; in such a case, the child, in his efforts to achieve the behaviour pattern expected of him, has warped his personal psychological development and the only expression of such abnormality may be the abnormal speech pattern. If the speech defect is a symptom of psychological maladjustment in the individual, as that individual's mental attitude changes, so will the symptom change.

Drawing and painting are here considered as a means through which a child's mental attitude may be changed, resulting in changes in the speech pattern and thereby treatment.

What kinds of drawings have therapeutic value?

The answer is: drawings that are recognizably symbols of the child's personal psychology and thus represent his inner attitude as it is at the time the drawing is done.

Is it natural for a child to produce such drawings?

I would say it is. Children are natural in themselves and are in touch with their own personal fantasy world and can express such fantasy freely and easily. They are not conscious of the fact that their fantasy is a symbol of their personal psychology, but that does not alter the fact that such is the case – this is recognized by all schools of depth psychology. Some psychologically disturbed children produce their personal fantasies naturally and spontaneously. The psychological maladjustment of other children may be associated with the fact that they are cut off from the fund of personal fantasy which should be natural to all children. In other cases of psychological maladjustment, the child knows the fantasies, but he dare not share these fantasies with others – he erects a barricade of some type to prevent himself from doing so.

If a child is unable to fantasy freely and naturally, what can the therapist do to help him in this matter?

The need is for the therapist to have a knowledge of the life of childhood and its development into mature adulthood. Necessary pre-requisites are: (1) the personal conviction that it is right and natural for fantasy to exist in all children; (2) the realization that this conviction can often be conveyed to a child without discussion, but by simply taking it for granted that the child can and will produce fantasy; (3) the realization that the child who has difficulty in producing fantasy must feel he can trust the therapist completely – he is likely to be trusting her with things which, to him, are precious personal secrets, sometimes secrets about which he feels guilty. Before trusting her, he may need to "sense" that the therapist has deep personal integrity and is sympathetic to his needs. If the child has such a relationship with the therapist, it does not seem to matter whether the therapist is a gentle person or a strong, robust sort of individual – the personality of the therapist will vary; (4) the realization that the child may produce ideas and concepts which are contrary to the therapist's own moral and possibly conventional outlook and that any criticism of his production, whether expressed by the therapist or sensed by the child, is likely to dam the spring which needs to flow if treatment is to be successful; (5) the realization that the most unimaginative-looking drawing may reveal an unexpected wealth of fantasy if appropriate questions are put to the child; for example, Does anyone live in the house? Are they there now? Where have they gone to? What is this? What is it doing? and so on.

To what extent does the child's drawing need to be consciously interpreted to him?

In my experience, conscious interpretation is not, necessarily, essential. Obviously the more insight and understanding the therapist has of the workings of the unconscious, the more will she be able to understand the symbolism of the drawings the child produces, both in relation to his own psychology and to his family's psychology; according to, and in the light of, the extent of her understanding, she will comment to the child and talk to the parent. In the absence of such understanding, the therapist's personal honesty, on which I have already commented, should make her acknowledge her lack of understanding to herself and should make her look upon the child and his drawing as a means through which she is going to be taught something. I have found that the therapist who has little or no knowledge of unconscious symbols, but whose approach to her patient has been that outlined under the points 1 to 5 enumerated above, has been able to receive a fund of fantasy from a child with extremely beneficial results both from the points of view of the child's psychology as a whole and of the speech pattern.

Can this line of approach be used with a group of children?
I would say No. Unless he is a child whose psychology is so grossly abnormal that the presence of others makes no difference to him, his productions are likely to be influenced to some extent by his personal reactions to others in the group and by what those others are doing. I would, myself, believe that the fantasy to which I have been referring is personal to the child only if it is produced with no person other than the therapist present.

Why should a change occur in a child's psychology, and in his symptom, through the sharing of his fantasy with an adult who wishes to help and understand him?
To understand this, one needs to accept the fact that an individual is made up of his unconscious as well as his conscious sides and to accept the fact that if there is maladjustment in the unconscious this is shown through abnormal symptoms appearing in conscious behaviour (I am using the word "behaviour" in the broadest sense of the term). Conscious behaviour is that which the outside world sees and of which a child can be made aware (although some children are not so aware unless their attention is drawn to their abnormal behaviour by other children or adults – for example, there are cases of young children who seem unaware of their stammer). The juxtaposition of the components within the unconscious and conscious needs to be one of harmony – otherwise maladjustment is present. As I have already said, all schools of depth psychology recognize that the personal fantasies expressed by children in their drawings are images of the unconscious. The unconscious when attempting to express itself in images seeks to find a solution to maladjustment. As a solution satisfactory to the whole personality is found, so a change occurs in conscious behaviour; the symptom of maladjustment is no longer necessary.

Here are some drawings produced by children, each of whom has been seen individually by a speech therapist – not necessarily myself – to substantiate the contention that the drawings mirror both the child's problem and its solution.

CASE I

As regards the first child, F.K., results of intelligence tests and school attainments showed that he was a boy of good average intelligence. The parents noticed a tendency to hesitate when speaking before he first went to school. This became marked soon after he was five. I saw him when he was six years nine months. Speech was not blocked but reiteration was persistent on sounds, syllables or whole words. *T* and *d* were substituted for *r* and *k* and no combinations of consonants were used. In view of the dyslalia and the persistent reiteration it was not always easy to understand the boy. He was the elder of two children, his sister being a year younger. The home was a good one. No member on either side of the family had had a speech problem nor did there seem to be any evidence of psychological maladjustment in members of the family. F.K. mixed easily with others; he had no marked fears; he was normally venturesome; he was getting on well in school. The only symptom, apart from the abnormal speech patterns, was that he seemed excessively immature for a normal little boy of nearly seven.

Here are the drawings which he made on the first occasion I saw him (p. 122).

DRAWING 1. There are two bulls. A large stone, pushed by a fox, has fallen on one bull and has broken a bone in its leg. The other bull is coming to help the injured bull.

I do not think anyone would quibble at the concept that bulls represent strong masculine elements. The drawings suggest that all is not well with the masculine element in F.K. but at least masculine help is at hand.

DRAWING 2 was done on the same day. A man is trying to step from one mountain to another. There is a dangerous drop into which he might "smash" himself – there is water below – the man dives into the water and is O.K. There is a horse belonging to the man which is escaping from the man. It is trying to find the water to get into it. It is scared of the water because there are sharks in

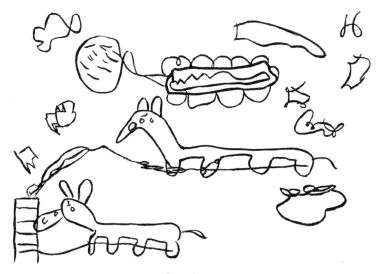

Drawing 1

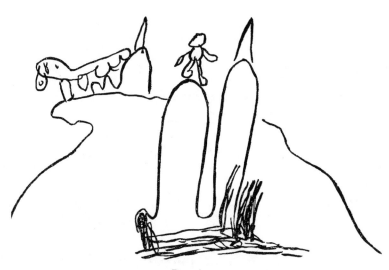

Drawing 2

it. F.K. called the man "Stephen Lawrence" and then changed this to "Stephen Betty".

I asked the mother about Stephen Lawrence and Stephen Betty. Stephen Lawrence proved to be the name of the boy who lived next door – a boy a year older than F.K. who, according to the mother, was "a very nice boy" but "a rough type". Stephen Betty is the thirteen-year-old son of the mother's sister Betty, also named Stephen, and called Stephen Betty by F.K. to differentiate him from Stephen Lawrence. This teenager was said by the mother to act as "father" and to be the authority for the younger children. Thus the man in the drawing would seem to represent a growing male, with a rougher and more adult personality than had, as yet, appeared in F.K. himself. This part of F.K. is shown to be in a serious predicament. The predicament is dealt with by the man diving into the water; an action which has no fears for him.

All schools of depth psychology recognize water as being symbolic of the unconscious. Before something new in a person's psychology materializes, frequently the concept of diving into, or being in, water is expressed. The horse, in symbolism, is often expressive of a life-giving force. In the drawing, the man (the male – the masculine) is separated from his horse (from his life-giving force). The horse, however, is trying to get to the place where he can join the man – he is afraid of getting into this water as it contains terrifying creatures. This is not unnatural because the animal instincts of all human beings contain elements which are naturally frightening and which need to be recognized and faced.

What I had been told about F.K., and the impression the boy had given me, was confirmed by these drawings. Both drawings indicated that all was not well with his masculine side. In real life his personality was still that of a baby rather than that of a nearly seven-year-old boy. These drawings, however, indicated that the masculine side of the boy was trying to find the solution in its own way.

Shortly afterwards, F.K. drew what he called a picture of "the sun rising and stretching". In symbolism the sun is recognized as being male. F.K. had expressed exactly what was happening – his maleness was rising and stretching.

His sister then began to appear in his drawings. She, although younger, had always been the more boyish and aggressive of the two children. As these more masculine aggressive characters, combined with feminine ones, appeared in his drawings, so did his own masculine side find its rightful place.

F.K. is now seven-and-a-half years old. His manner, his stance, his attitude in general are now those of a boy and not those of an immature, young child. As this state of affairs has developed, the stammer has decreased. Combined consonants have established themselves spontaneously. The k and t, g and d substitutions are subsiding but the standard patterns are not yet fully established.

CASE II

The next drawings were done by an eight-year-old girl. She was an extremely bossy, domineering child. She was unpopular at school because she interfered with and organized everyone. The stammer was first heard shortly after the inception of speech. When first seen at the clinic, just before her eighth birthday, her speech was handicapped by persistent blocking of a moderate nature. Intelligence tests and school attainments indicated that J.C. was of average intelligence. The mother was a vague, not very intelligent person who had no grip on anything. The only other child, a boy four years younger, was completely out of hand; the mother seemed quite surprised that people saw this child in that light. It never seemed to dawn on her that she should control him. The father, too, was an ineffectual person. He provided well for his family's material needs but he took no personal interest in his children and made no attempt to control them. Thus neither child was given any help in learning to control or make profitable creative use of their over-abundant aggression.

DRAWING 1. This drawing was done just before J.C's eighth birthday. J.C. is in bed. "Black Men" (her term) are coming through the window to kill her.

This drawing represents J.C's psychology as a whole at that time. J.C., the little girl, is in bed; she is not out and about in the world. The masculine aspects of J.C. are black and dangerous towards the little girl part of herself. This dangerously aggressive side is associated with the outside world (where J.C's aggression showed) and it is going to kill the little-girl side of herself. The therapist understood

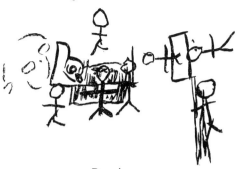

Drawing 1

what was happening and realized that there was no hope of getting the parents to understand and help the child in her predicament. She realized that the child needed to be helped to develop her feminine (little-girl) side. She also realized that the unconscious was likely to be as strong in feminine elements as it was in masculine elements, if only J.C. were given an opportunity to let her unconscious express itself. J.C. was therefore encouraged to produce further drawings so that unconscious images could come to the fore, while, at the same time, she was encouraged to become interested in feminine pursuits.

The following drawing was done just before she was discharged, thirteen months later.

DRAWING 2. This drawing exemplifies the contention that a drawing may look very "ordinary", but may prove to contain far more ideas than appear on the surface. On being asked about the picture, the child told the therapist that a wise old man and a wise old woman leave the house to collect wood. The other man finds the tree and climbs it. There is a nest at the top with an egg in it. The wise old man suggests they keep the egg, but the wise old woman says, "No, it is not our egg; it is the bird's mother's. She has laid it and there is another little bird in it." So they let the egg stay in the nest so that another little bird may hatch.

The female bird had laid the egg which is now being allowed to grow and develop. The tree in which the growth is to take place could well be the symbol for the tree of life.

The child had ceased to draw symbols of the aggression which had

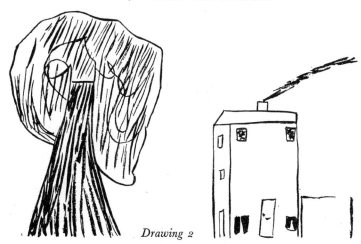

Drawing 2

been killing her female side. During the thirteen months following the first drawing there entered her productions the ideas of finding new things, small girls playing, and the idea such as is expressed in this drawing. Her feminine side was no longer being killed, it was developing. Her aggressive masculine side was achieving a position more in proportion to a girl's personality. As this change occurred, she ceased to be so bossy – she became interested in knitting and cooking, she became more feminine; the speech pattern also changed, speech became fluent and easy.

CASE III

This example shows how an environment and upbringing which convention considers excellent may be adversely affecting a child's psychology.

H.D. was a very intelligent boy. Everyone spoke most highly of his parents. They had been born in one of the worst localities of London's East End and each had had an extremely hard childhood. H.D's mother had when a child been used as a little drudge; she had been led to believe that her own mother was an ailing woman who must not lift a finger – this old lady is now eighty and still has her eighty-two-year-old husband at her beck and call. The mother had loathed the crudeness, the squalor and the hardness of

East End life. When H.D's father was a baby, his mother had died. His father was a brutal man. H.D's father and his sister had, when children, left their own father and had taken a room on their own as soon as the boy left school at fourteen. They had their mother's wedding ring and they survived by pawning it at the beginning of each week to buy food and redeeming it again at the end of the week with their earnings.

It was hard to realize that these parents came from such backgrounds. They were a well-dressed, well-spoken, kindly, appreciative, intelligent pair. Their desire was to forget their roots and see to it that their children should never experience the roughness and hardness they had experienced. They had moved into West Kent in order to get away from their East End environment. Although these parents were giving H.D. and their elder son an excellent, sensible, affectionate home life, the boy reacted to me as though he were a deprived child, when seen at the age of five years five months. I use the word "deprived" as it is used by those who are responsible for children who, for one reason or another, have experienced broken unhappy homes. Frequently these children show traits of their insecurity long after they have been found foster mothers or have become members of a children's home. They come up to strangers in a pathetic manner, obviously asking for approval and affection and wanting to be noticed, they give you something which belongs to them in order to make contact with you, and so on. H.D. reacted in this way to me. He had stammered since the age of two and a half years. The stammer had taken the form of tense repetition of syllables.

DRAWING 1. The child said about this drawing, "The horse has a little house on its head; the horse doesn't like this. A man lives in the house and grows cabbages on the horse's back. He makes spells on the horse with the help of a witch. The buffalo is the horse's friend. He eats the house, man and the cabbages and butts the witch, and so the horse is freed."

DRAWING 2. The following drawing, which was done a week later, is on the same theme. "The good goblin goes to the help of the horse who wants to be free of the house on its head. The goblin makes the horse sit cross-legged and then sits on the horse's hind legs till the house slips off. The horse then prances around."

SIGNS, SIGNALS AND SYMBOLS

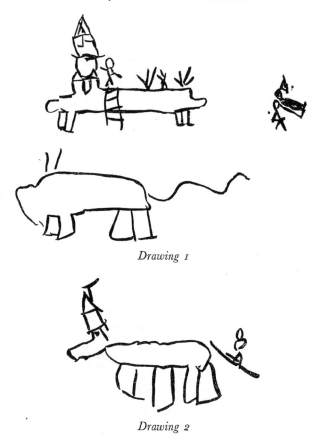

Drawing 1

Drawing 2

The house is a neat, tidy, well-kept house. It is like the house in which H.D's mother is bringing him up. It has a garden in the first drawing, as does his home. The house bears no resemblance to the rough East End gardenless homes of his grandparents. The drawings say that the neat tidy house is being cast off in order that H.D's own life force (the horse) may be freed.

The parents wanted to obliterate their roots; they wanted to bring up their children as though their roots did not exist. They were not developing their children's lives from these roots; they were trying to cover up those roots by superimposing something which was more acceptable to them.

After freeing his life force from the house that the parents were trying to make him carry, the boy drew a picture which contained a baby in a pram. A new child was developing. The new child was a little tough rough East Ender. The brutality and crudeness, however, which the parents had known, were redeemed through all the good, positive features which did exist in their desires for their children. The child himself helped the mother to see that she had been attempting to superimpose on him something which was unsuitable for him. On one occasion she called the boy in for tea after seeing an older boy take H.D's cap and throw it away. As the child (then not yet six) came in he said, "You shouldn't have done that, Mum. Tea's not ready. I was doing all right." This sort of experience helped her to see that her desire to keep him from anything remotely associated with crudeness, hardness and brutality was causing her to be dishonest, as well as expecting him to form into a mould which was unsuitable for him. As the child cast off all that was associated with preventing him from experiencing the hard rock-bottom instinctual facts of life, he ceased to have the manner of a deprived child. His birthright was no longer being turned into something which it was not; he became a real little "tough guy" and the stammer decreased.

Summary and conclusion

A child's drawing may symbolize his psychological situation at the time the drawing is done. An abnormal speech pattern may be *the*, or one of the, outward sign(s) of psychological maladjustment. When psychological maladjustment exists, a child's drawings may express, in symbolic form, the nature of that maladjustment and its solution. The drawing of images referring to the latter has been found to coincide with the integration of the personality of the child. The psychological maladjustment being resolved, its outward signs are mitigated.

I want to thank my speech therapy colleagues, Miss Ellis, Mrs France and Miss Umpleby, for giving me the opportunity to see their cases and for allowing me to use drawings, some of which were done while the child concerned was being seen by one of them and some of which were done during the child's interview with me.

REFERENCES

Fordham, M. (1947) *The Life of Childhood*, London, Kegan Paul
Fordham, M. (1957) *New Developments in Analytical Psychology*, London, Routledge
Jung, C. G. (1919) *The Psychology of the Unconscious*, London, Kegan Paul
Jung, C. G. (1945) *Modern Man in Search of a Soul*, London, Kegan Paul
Jung, C. G. (1953) *Psychology of Alchemy* **12** in *Collected Works*, London, Routledge
Jung, C. G. (1953) *Two Essays on Analytical Psychology* **7** in *Collected Works*, London, Routledge
Jung and Kerényi (1951) *Introduction to a Science of Mythology*, London, Routledge
Wickes Frances (1943) *The Inner World of Childhood*, New York and London, Appleton Century

14

STELLA E. MASON, Birmingham

Informative and Manipulative Signs and Signals in Language Disorder

This contribution aims to be an unbiased approach to the problem of the diagnosis and treatment of a language disorder hitherto included under the heading "dyslalia". In the case presented a full description of the language used by the patient is not given, for the concern is the dynamic structure of the speaker, the context and the motivation of his speech deviations.

The criterion of "bad or "difficult" speech is employed by many authors for the grouping of types of articulation regarded as disordered, defective or retarded, as in Van Riper's "articulatory disorder" (1950) and the authorized definition of the College of Speech Therapists (1959). Hence the term "dyslalia" derived from *dys* – "badly, with difficulty" and *laleo* – "I speak". It would appear that these authorities are giving the concept of articulation primary value. Yet other writers, notably Jespersen (1922), Lewis (1947), Stein (1942, 1949), and lately Epstein (1960), take a different view. Jespersen, Seth and Guthrie (1935) and earlier writers such as Steinthal (1881) draw attention to the fact that in infancy one can find a wide range of so-called primordial sounds. Later the child will not use some of these sounds even when they occur in the mother tongue; others occur in some languages, particularly primitive ones. Lewis (1951) points out that a speech sound "has not absolute value, once and for all, but that its effectiveness in action depends upon its relationship to the other sounds with which it forms a pattern". Stein (1953) puts forward the idea that so-called basic "articulatory" patterns are genetically fixed and that they have to be evaluated in relation to those of the community.

Briefly, the rudimentary beginnings of speech in an infant may be said to consist in a growth of modes of action related to such pleasurable activities as sucking, chewing, vocalizing and so on. These become integrated into a pattern of behaviour and when the infant attaches referential value to certain sound-combinations he is making use of language; when the institution "language" becomes the activity called speaking, verbal communication takes place by means of a codified system of signs, signals and symbols, the function being to "influence the course and determine the nature of relationships". The instrumental uses of spoken conventional words have been given the terms "declarative" and "manipulative" by Lewis (1947, 1951).

Professor Lewis (1951) considers that "the chief clue to understanding the development of the child's speech lies in considering the situations in which it is used"; that "progress consists not in learning words as names labelling or representing things but in the growth of power to use vocal behaviour as a means of supplementing – and in the end, replacing – other behaviour" (1951). Although this refers to the development of so-called normal, standard or accepted speech, it should be equally useful to use the same frame of reference in order to discover what lies behind the development of so-called abnormal, non-standard speech. This is illustrated in the following case.

Case history

The patient was a boy aged five who was described as "having speech that was at times unintelligible". Hearing ability and intelligence appeared satisfactory, there was no orthodontic abnormality. The boy's personality appeared on first acquaintance to be reasonably well adjusted – he gave the impression of being a happy, eager-to-please though rather shy boy. No specific incidents in the boy's history indicating physical or emotional trauma have been elicited.

Features of speech

The outstanding feature in spontaneous speech noted during the first interview was that there was apparently no consistency in the sound changes. For instance, instead of "Are you having strawberries for tea?", he said "Are you habing tawbeid por tea?" and for "Is someone else having strawberries?", he said "Id lomewone elt habing pawbei?" From this sample, which is typical of his speech at that time, it is seen that, for instance, s changes variously into l, t, p or zero. There is, however, no "speech defect" in the sense of current terminology, for there are no defective articulatory sounds, nor is there anything wrong with the ability to articulate. He can articulate with the facility of any standard speaker. What observation shows is merely that he uses words in a form not contained in the English vocabulary. He may be said to have a language of his own. His idiolect is in an extreme statistical minority and "abnormal" only in this sense.

Therapeutic procedure

The first two or three interviews naturally were spent in establishing a relationship with the therapist and her consulting rooms, during which time he maintained his original patterns of language and behaviour. After a few weeks his behaviour underwent a sudden and remarkable change. The shy boy became noisy, destructive, physically violent and verbally threatening. Since there are many clues regarding the personality of the child and his conflicts contained in these threats, it is appropriate to quote some of them here with proffered interpretations. They are quoted verbatim though no attempt is made to reproduce the actual pronunciation.

"When I go home I'll go into my room and do some magic and in the morning you'll feel all queer."

This threat marked the onset of the sudden change in the boy's behaviour and showed overtly his need to control the environment. In the treatment situation the patient projects unconscious images on the therapist. As all relationships stem from the basic relationship with the mother (Neumann, 1955) it can be assumed that the therapist takes the part of, that is, she is identified with the mother. The dark side of the mother is full of magical, terrifying powers and it is natural to deal with fear of an object by becoming that object, for in this way it is possible to become as terrifying as the object itself. Thus by turning the tables and using magic himself the boy can destroy the idea of the mother's phallic magic, showing that there are greater powers than she. His recognition and acknowledgment of the aspect of the Terrible Mother and her powers was made clear when the therapist misquoted the boy. He said "I don't do bad magic, I do good magic. You do bad magic."

"I'm going to put golden syrup in your eyes and wee-wee and motion on it and stick a sword right through your eyes, then you won't be able to see."

The sticky substance of golden syrup together with urine and faeces, all powerful magic tools, as shown by many anthropologists (Douglas, M., 1955) (Sumner, H. G., 1947), are here being used to overthrow the therapist, who is becoming dangerous and seeing too much.

That the boy is unconsciously trying to find the solution to his problem seems to be corroborated by the following fantasy:

"I'm going to turn a key in you, then I shall see all inside you. Nobody can see inside me. Now I'm turning the key – horrible, horrible, horrible."

His preoccupation with keys, for he is fascinated by them, indicates his realization of the twofold function of a key. It is used to lock and keep things secret, safe and hidden, and to unlock and reveal what has so far been hidden. Keys may keep one out or let one in. The boy wants to have his cake and eat it. He wants to see what is hidden from him yet does not want to reveal his own secrets. He knows that what is locked up (the unconscious, Pandora's box containing every human ill) is horrible and he fears to look and yet is fascinated by the sexual aspect of his own "horrible" shadow. The key and the lock are well-known sexual symbols (Partridge, 1949, s.v.).

This boy not only signalled his distress verbally as in the above examples but in other ways also. A typical drawing gives a further indication of his desperate attempts to work out his ambivalence to the mother-figure who is unpredictable and can be good and bad at the same time.

DRAWING 1. The squiggles are apparently magical emanations and he makes it clear that magic can be performed by urine. He also emphasizes that his phallus is much more powerful than that of the therapist. "That's you doing a wee-wee and this is me doing an *enormous* wee-wee." The urine that his own phallus produces bears also a resemblance to a snake and the magic arms and legs

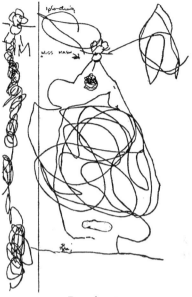

Drawing 1

given to the therapist are reminiscent of the many-armed goddesses typified in Indian folklore. That the two figures of the patient himself and the therapist are expressions of *unconscious* figures that overpower him seems to be clear when contrasted with the tiny figure drawn at the bottom of the page which he said was "a creature that no one has ever seen before and those things (the horizontal lines) are to steady it". It appears to be the patient himself as he really is in contrast to his fantasy image. He draws a picture of his own still powerless ego.

His choice of symbolic signalling may be further illustrated by a drawing he made at a later stage of treatment.

DRAWING 2. The therapist was first drawn with six legs and wings. When it was pointed out to him that he had made her half bad because she had lots of legs like a spider and half good because she had angel's wings, he drew a fire which "burnt her all up". The "fire" was at first drawn over the legs and when he was shown that he had burnt or destroyed only her bad qualities he scribbled a little

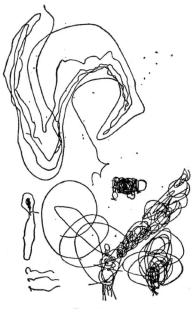

Drawing 2

more over the figure then drew a maze, saying as he did so, "I wonder how I'm going to get out of this".

Interpretations of the kind that are given here were naturally not always offered to the boy, but interpretations of a kind that could be understood by him and were not too shattering were given and on each occasion appeared to afford him immediate relief. For instance, when it was said, "I think you're killing me so that you can kill all the bad secret things in yourself", he answered, "You're quite right, quite right", and became demonstratively affectionate. Sometimes he offered his own interpretations. On one occasion he spent some time sticking matches into the therapist's arm. When he was asked why he wanted to hurt her he said, "I like you too much". Again, when the therapist asked why she was being killed, he said, "When I was your friend, a long time ago, I said something to you and you didn't understand and it hurt me, it hurt me very much".

Diagnosis

Some situations in which the speech abnormalities of the patient occurred have been mentioned. It remains to make an attempt to understand the nature of his speech. It emerged that what might be described as his disordered articulation was used as a signalling code. During one visit there was such a marked deterioration in his speech that attention was drawn to it by the therapist. He said "I don't want to top coming eber" (I don't want to stop coming, ever). He was asked if he was afraid that if his speech improved he would have to stop coming and he replied "Yet" (Yes). It was suggested that if his speech didn't improve it might be considered that there was no point in his visits being continued. He made no direct reply but said, "I think I'll put the lights on in the doll's house" – and his articulation of this sentence was correct. This seemingly disjointed remark showed that "the light shineth in the darkness" – that is, the motive became conscious.

In order to understand a system of signs, signals and symbols it is necessary for both the sender and the receiver to understand the code. In a language disorder it is likely that the listener is not in possession of the code (speech is unintelligible) but it is also possible that the speaker himself may not be fully aware of his secret code. In sharing the standard code of signs and symbols of the community in which he lives, the informative aspect of language is brought into use. Yet words cloak as well as clothe ideas (Stein 1953), and as a means of dealing with the environment the manipulative aspect of language takes precedence. In manipulating the environment one does not necessarily have knowledge of the motives behind the manipulation. The patient finds himself in a situation where the use of a secret code is imperative, yet he may not be conscious of the key to his own code: he knows the superficial meanings of the words he uses but he does not understand his own secret.

What is this boy's secret? The answer may lie in the fact that, in this case as in others, an abnormality in the child-mother relationship is likely to result in anxiety and veiled aggression and forms the basis of all future relationships. It is these emotional factors, anxiety and veiled aggression, by necessity repressed and therefore unrecognized, that may account for the secrecy.

The child does not say, "I wish to be loved as I need to be loved. I want you to treat me as the baby I should like to be and am behaving as though I am, as you can see by the way I speak." He *dare* not say, "I hate you for being a witch and denying me the love that I consider is my right", and so both in his behavioural and in his verbal language he must deal with his situation as best he can. His overwhelming feelings result in an urge to talk, yet what he says and the manner of his speech must, for safety's sake, disguise his hidden wishes and forbidden anger. He may obtain relief and even pleasure or triumph in the use of his secret code in the same way that Ferreira (1960) suggests the schizophrenic obtains relief in language. First, to speak at all is an act of appeasement in cases where silence would call forth anger and punishment. Secondly, there is pleasure in a self-assertive action and a feeling of triumph over the listener by sending a message that cannot be understood. Thirdly, criticism can be expressed without fear. This is reminiscent of the motives behind the creation of secret languages characteristic of adolescent years.

To remove from such a patient his powerful tools by giving him "articulation exercises" and the like, and thereby removing his language disorder, is perhaps to do him a grave disservice for he will have to find some other way of giving vent to his feelings. Other psychosomatic symptoms might arise which, though they might not be of such an obvious type, could well cause greater suffering. The patient who speaks in a secret code does not communicate his thoughts, for in fact he much fears to be understood. Thus an added terror sets in: the fear that the code be broken and the hidden feelings made public. Such treatment cannot in truth be called successful. The therapist's remedial approach must depend on true diagnosis, for treatment guided by a classification made by means of inappropriate criteria, even if seemingly effective, is most likely to be harmful to the patient's personality structure.

In disorders of the kind exemplified there are two languages in use, one consisting of words used in the cultural group, the other consisting of a system of individual and personal signs, signals and symbols. One language runs along and is contrary to the other, hence it would be preferable to make use of the Greek prefix *para* – "beside" – in the coining of the diagnostic term. The introduction of the term *rhema* and the account given of its meaning and use[1] make it undeniable that, semantically, this word most nearly and accurately fulfils the function demanded of it. It is therefore suggested that certain cases of language disorder should be classified as *pararhetic* and the disorder should be known as *pararhesis*. This definition adequately marks the distinction between such disorders of language described here and cases where the term dyslalia can be corroborated.

Members of our discipline would not then trick themselves and others by applying correct logic to a term which may have either a descriptive or a diagnostic meaning and so run the risk of arriving at a notion that is as stringent and absurd as saying that if no cat has two tails and one cat has one more tail than no cat, one cat must have three tails.

REFERENCES

Douglas, Mary (1955) "The Social and Religious Symbolisms of the Lele of the Kasai". *Zaïre* IX/4

Epstein, A. G. (1960) "Phonemic Testing", *Journal of the South African Logopedic Society*

Ferreira, Antonio J. (1960) "The Semantics and the Context of the Schizophrenic's Language", *Archives of General Psychiatry* **3**

Jespersen, Otto (1922) *Language. Its Nature, Development and Origin*, London, Allen and Unwin

Lewis, M. M. (1947) *Language in Society*, London, Nelson

Lewis, M. M. (1951) *Infant Speech*, London, Routledge

Neumann, E. (1955) *The Great Mother*, Routledge

Partridge, Eric (1949) *Dictionary of Slang*, 3rd ed., London, Routledge

Seth, G., and Guthrie, D. (1935) *Speech in Childhood*, Oxford University Press

Stein, L. (1942) *Speech and Voice*, London, Methuen

Stein, L. (1949) *The Infancy of Speech and the Speech of Infancy*, London, Methuen

Stein, L. (1953) "Stammering as a Psychosomatic Disorder", *Folia Phoniatrica* **5**, No. 1

[1] See Chapter 2.

Steinthal, H. (1881) *Abriss Der Sprachwissenschaft*, Berlin, Dümmler

Sumner, H. G., Keller, A. G., Davie, M. R. (1947) *The Science of Society*, 5th ed., Yale University Press

Terminology for Speech Pathology, College of Speech Therapists, London (1959)

Van Riper, C. (1950) *Speech Correction*, New York, Prentice – Hall

15

R. E. SIMMS, Nottingham

The Data Underlying the Concept of Dyslalia

It is necessary to define roughly the term dyslalia as it is used in the three following reports of findings undertaken as a joint project, in order to show clearly the type of case to be described. There is much variation in the use of this word. People are guided by different concepts in describing particular cases, therefore they arrive at different definitions. The fact that they all use the same term then leads us to believe there is only one concept of dyslalia. The result is that we have to define and re-define terms each time a paper is written, and it seems that for speech pathology the accuracy should be questioned when so few therapists are agreed on the extent of the field to which the term dyslalia applies.

We appear to become side-tracked into listing causes rather than describing the speech of our patients. People seem to be perturbed by the many causes of the same disorder, but it would seem that it is because they confuse cause with reason or factor. For instance, the fall of a tile from a roof may be caused by a high wind or a careless tiler, but the factor or reason for the fall is gravity.

In the current terminology dyslalia is given as "defects of articulation or slow development of articulatory patterns" – with a description of the defect as we know it. These defective articulatory patterns may be caused by deficient intelligence, emotional disturbance, immaturity or the imitation of abnormal patterns of articulation. In passing, I would comment on the given causes and say that deficient intelligence may cover anything from an I.Q. of

80 to zero, so that even the speech of an imbecile may be known as dyslalic.

Children who constantly associate with persons who suffer from defective speech – caused for example by partial deafness, neurological defects or cleft palate – may imitate the speech and acquire the defect themselves, but others in very similar situations do not. It may be assumed that there are some predisposing factors apart from the obvious conditions which enable one child to acquire an adequate speech system in the face of many difficulties and prevent another in a similar situation from doing the same.

There are apparently only few examples of this type of imitation; one case is known of a child who had, on the face of it, imitated her mother, a woman of very low intelligence whose speech was almost unintelligible. On detailed investigation it was found that the child's speech had not the same pattern as her mother's, and as the child, too, was of low intelligence it is likely that the speech condition would have been present in the child even if the speech of her mother had been normal. In the cases under consideration there were no factors of this kind to consider.

The children whose cases we have investigated show no overt signs of emotional disturbance and no physical signs of immaturity or maldevelopment, with the exception of so-called immaturity of speech. We feel, however, that there is room for more detailed investigation in this field.

Under the heading of *articulation* the official terminology mentions two terms, Sigmatism and Rhotacism, which are said to be descriptive but to have no aetiological connotations. It could be tentatively suggested that this consideration also applies to the term dyslalia, and that for this reason we must be very careful when we label a child dyslalic. It is quite harmless to name a group dyslalia and to place in it, perhaps temporarily as far as diagnosis is concerned, many questionable cases, but danger arises in the subsequent tendency to use the same method of treatment for all cases within the group.

Morley says that in the group dyslalia "there have been included those defects of articulation which appear to be functional in origin rather than attributable to any damage of the brain or failure of the neurological maturation for speech. In many there is spontaneous improvement or rapid response to guidance and treatment" (Morley, 1957). If the response is not rapid in a child who has been diagnosed as dyslalic, is it only suggested after treatment has failed that he is probably not dyslalic? In which group is he then placed? Allowing for the inevitable margin of error, a more accurate and far-seeing diagnosis would have been desirable and this is what we hope to achieve after further work along these lines.

Speech therapists are trained to adhere to a system or formula in the treatment of dyslalics and at the same time are reminded to treat the person, not the defect. In the treatment of so-called dyslalics one is left with a residue of cases who have not responded in the way that one would have expected. It is to these cases we now turn who, having had negative reports from audiologist, neurologist and psychologist, still fail to respond to the formula which has been worked out for them.

The current sound tests are too limited to *test*, or do not analyse the individual speech satisfactorily. Treatment depending on such tests will be similarly inadequate. In many textbooks the position in the word of the omitted or defective sound is considered to be of great importance. The tests consist of words in which a specific sound occurs initially, medially, or finally and the treatment follows the same pattern. We are advised to "teach" one sound at a time, first initially, because it is "easiest", then finally, then medially. The choice of the first sound to be taught is frequently taken at random. We are told that it is better to teach first the sounds *b*, *p* and *m*, because the patient can *see* them being made. This may help the patient a great deal, but even if it does, it seems to imply that auditory discrimination is at fault and should, therefore, be replaced by visual perception, an assumption which is not always tenable. It is said that *initial* sounds are taught first because they are easiest. For whom, the patient or the therapist? It saves a considerable amount of time if patients find the same things easy and the same things difficult but, unfortunately, this is not so. There does not seem to be a sufficiently good reason in many cases for teaching an "easy" sound first. Shames and Fisher, in their report on the relationship of types of articulation errors to intelligibility of speech (1960), say that as a result of their study it is felt that therapy for children having multiple articulation errors should be directed towards those sounds most highly related to intelligibility (and that frequency of appearance may be only one of the criteria for the selection of a sound for improvement).

When the patient is able to articulate the individual sound he is then taught to use it in words, then in short sentences, then in stories, rhymes, and word games where it is, or should be, used spontaneously. Having achieved this, the sound is learnt at the ends of words and when, at last, he can use it in the middle of words he sets out to learn the next sound.

If the patient has not started to use the sound in *all* positions in spontaneous speech to an ever-increasing extent all the time he has been learning it, he is not likely to start using it in spontaneous speech when *we* consider he is ready to do so, and have been led to believe he would. Why should it be so difficult to bridge the gap between exercises in the book and general spontaneous conversation with a child who has "kept pace with the formula" until this point? It appears that while the patient accepts instruction and correction when applied to isolated words, phrases and sentences, in fact, in exercises far removed from ordinary speech, he is unable to accept instruction and correction when it interferes with his meaningful language – the expression of his thoughts and narrative description.

While it is true to say that many experienced speech therapists, realizing the inadequacy of this system, have abandoned it in favour of more suitable procedures, many newly qualified therapists are constantly baffled by their apparent failure in the treatment of what they had expected to be the least complicated of speech disorders. In time they will either work out their own tests and treatment procedures or they will find that they are following no system at all, but changing their ideas and opinions with each so-called "dyslalic" who comes to the clinic.

Our considerations led to an investigation of the structure of the language of "dyslalic" children, and for the purposes of investigation we had to collect data which could be subjected to phonemic analysis. This was not a simple matter for we needed to record an example of absolutely spontaneous speech, suitable in length and substance, from one of our selected cases.

Robert, the boy we chose for our project, is aged eight and has an I.Q. of 96 on the Terman Merrill Scale. He had been attending the speech clinic for about two years. He is the fourth of five children of an average family and no other member has any speech defect. He shows no signs of neurological defect or hearing loss and there is nothing in his background to suggest emotional disturbance; he is friendly, though a little shy and normally mischievous. He suffered no birth injury, there were no feeding difficulties, in fact no evidence can be found of any abnormality in development with the exception of speech. His school work, though handicapped by his speech, is reported to be average, he has difficulty with reading but his arithmetic is good. He is able to produce any sound in isolation and most sounds in simple words, by imitation. His spontaneous speech, to the stranger, is unintelligible.

For the purpose of investigation we needed suitable test material that would evoke spontaneous speech without need of the written word or any spoken guidance on the part of the therapist. To find such material proved to be very difficult. All the available picture stories were either too long or too short, most of them required reading ability and many of them were not clear or simple enough for the child to understand; this necessitated explanation on the part of the therapist and therefore defeated the purpose. Eventually a book that met our requirements was found (Möller-Nielsen). It is a simple story in big, clear pictures of an adventure of a fish. The children understand the pictures and have no difficulty in working out the story.

In choosing Robert's recording we were influenced by the fact that it is short, and although this has disadvantages, other factors made this recording one of the most suitable for the purpose of the pilot investigation.

Robert had never seen the book before the recording used for analysis was made, and so he had no idea what to expect and had no guidance in any way from the therapist. This is the story as he told it when looking at the following pictures.

SIGNS, SIGNALS AND SYMBOLS

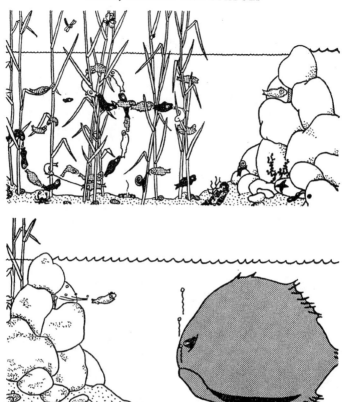

#wɔn	ˈdeɪ	ə	ˈfɪʔ(s)	ˈwɛn
one	day	a	fish	went
fʊu	ə	ˈʔoʊl#	#ˈʔɪ	ˈʔɪ
through	a	hole.	He	he
wɛnt	ˈfʊu	ən	sɔː	ə
went	through	and	saw	a
ˈbrɪ̥	ˈbrɪ̥	ˈʋɛ	ˈfɪɪ̥#	#də
big	big	red	fish.	The

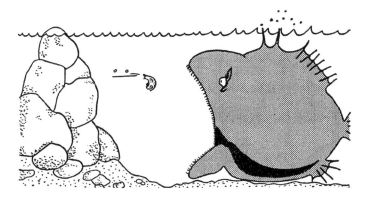

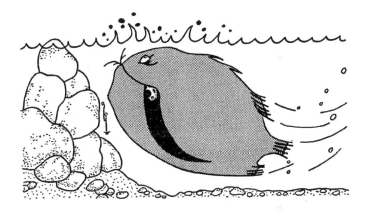

'bɪ	'ʊɛ	'fɪỹ	'wɛntə	dɛʔɪm
big	red	fish	went to	get him

i	'təm̄	'ʊaʊm#	#də	'bɪ
he	turn(ed)	round.	The	big

'ʊɛ	'fɪ	tsɔʔɪm#	#h'i	'm
red	fish	got (?stopped) him.	He	m

SIGNS, SIGNALS AND SYMBOLS

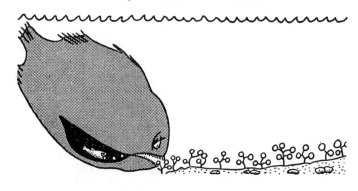

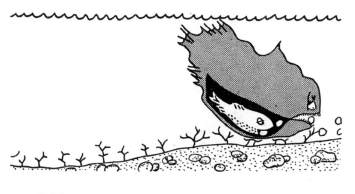

buḅɫ	ʔə	noʊ#	#'i	ðə
?	er	no.	He,	the
'brɨ̃	'frɨ̃	vɔɨ̃	'itɪn	ænd
big	fish	was	eating	and
ðəɪ	'wɛn	'ɪntu	ɪd̥	'maʊ
they	went	into	his	mouth
æn	'ɪntʊ	'du	də	'lɪʔɫ
and	into	?	the	little

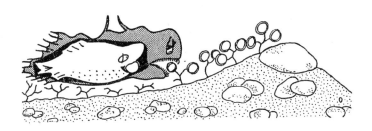

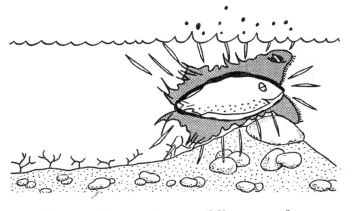

| 'fɪ# | #dɛn | də | 'lɪʔɫ | fɪ |
| fish. | Then | the | little | fish |

| dɔʔ | 'bɪɣ̃ə | æm | 'bɪʔə# | |
| got | bigger | and | bigger. | |

| #ən | 'soʊ | 'tsoʊ | i | ʋæm |
| And | so | so | he | ran |

| 'aʊt# | #ə | ʔɪ | naʊ# | #ən |
| out | of | his | mouth. | And |

SIGNS, SIGNALS AND SYMBOLS

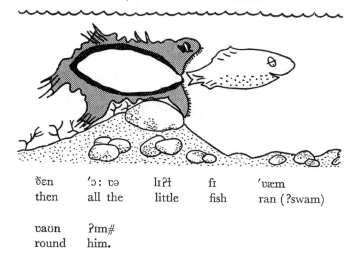

ðɛn	ˈɔː ʋə	lɪʔɬ	fɪ	ˈʋæm
then	all the	little	fish	ran (?swam)

ʋaʊn	ʔɪm#
round	him.

In this transcription IPA phonetic symbols are used whenever applicable. γ̊ most nearly resembles voiceless γ. ̪ under any symbol denotes a dental position.

The symbol # has been adopted from linguistics. "Silence or break in the sequence of elements will be indicated by #" (Harris, Z. S., 1957, p. 15).

To make a phonetic transcription of the recording was not a straight-forward matter because Robert uses a certain number of non-English sounds but three members of the research group agreed that it is as correct as possible at that point. Minor mistakes in phonetic transcription are not considered to be very important at this stage – since it is possible to check and correct the transcription in the later stages of phonemic analysis, when the language system begins to appear.

The transcription provides a corpus or stock of recorded utterances and a tape recording makes reference possible. These phonetic data provide the raw material which is to be subjected to a phonemic analysis so as to bring order into seemingly unconnected features, that is, to reveal the language *system* of the patient, which in its turn may be conducive to a truly diagnostic statement.

REFERENCES

Morley, M. E. (1957) *Development and Disorders of Speech in Childhood*, Edinburgh, Livingstone

Shames, G., and Fisher, J. (1960) "The Relationship of Types of Articulation Errors to Intelligibility of Speech", *Proc. XI Congress of Logopedics and Phoniatrics* (London 1959) Basle, Karger, *Speech* (1960) April

Möller-Nielsen, Egon. *Historie om Fisken*, Stockholm, Raben & Sjögren Bok-Förlag

Terminology for Speech Pathology (1959), College of Speech Therapists, London

Harris, Z. S. (1957) *Methods in Structural Linguistics*, University of Chicago Press, 3rd ed.

16

L. M. HARTLEY, Nottingham

Analysis of the Linguistic Data of Dyslalia

In turning towards the science of linguistics for an answer to the problem of dyslalia we were influenced by awareness of two main points. First, the dyslalic has a language of his own, a form of speech which is unique to him; secondly, the acquisition of language is a formidable task which can be accomplished only if all the mental faculties of the child continue working in close harmony.

As the foreigner cannot repeat sounds of an unfamiliar language that do not fit into his phonemic system, so it is not always easy to repeat the unintelligible speech of the dyslalic. We became aware that neither our phonemic system fitted into that of the dyslalic, nor his into ours; in other words, our phonemic systems are foreign to each other. On the assumption that the dyslalic has a language of his own it is important for the purpose of assessment to listen to it as though it were a meaningless jumble, as one does when listening to an unknown foreign language, rather than trying to distinguish complete and isolated words occurring one after the other, for "it must be remembered that speech is a set of complex continuous events, talking does not consist of separate sounds enunciated in succession" (Harris, 1951). It is very difficult to refrain from comparing how a dyslalic speaks with how one thinks he should speak. However, with practice attention may be paid to the content of the utterance as a whole rather than to sounds as though they are merely distortions of standard English speech. It also appears that in order to study a child's language it is of value to analyse it phonemically, that is, to examine the relationships between the sound units of the system and consequently find out the structure of the language. In other words, to diagnose rather than to rely on mere perception.

In making the phonemic analysis, the corpus (sample) was first divided into eight utterances. An utterance is "any stretch of talk by one person, before or after which there is silence on the part of the person. It is not in general identical with the sentence" (Harris, 1951). Juncture marks were placed where Robert took a breath.

The utterances were then divided into syllables such as CVC (C = Consonant, V = Vowel) as in /wən/ or CV as in /bi/. Stress and vowels occurring in a peak of prominence helped to determine the syllables. Sounds which may have begun or ended a syllable were termed interludes such as the /t/ of /wentə/.

The next step was to break down the syllables into phones, that is, into single speech sounds. We at first assumed all phones must be phonemes whereas we now know a phoneme is "a group of similar or related speech sounds which function analogously in a given language" (Harris, 1951). For example the features which distinguish "p" are its voiceless, bilabial and plosive qualities and only "p" has these three qualities. It is from the distinctive features that we can tell whether the phone is a phoneme or an allophone. An allophone is a member or variant of a phoneme; an example in our language is heard in the "t" in /stick/ and the "t" in /tick/. Therefore, an attempt was made to find from the distinctive features of the phones how many phonemes or allophones Robert had acquired in his language structure. This was done by examining his vowel system acoustically against his own dialectal background. Nothing unusual was observed either in his simple or diphthongal vowel systems. The consonants were put into the following categories:

Voice-Voiceless: e.g. /b/, /p/.
Position: e.g. velar or alveolar position /k/, /t/.
Obstruction: e.g. fricative or plosive /w/, /b/.

The phones were put into these three categories only to make it easier to describe the sound units and consequently find out whether to regard them as phonemes or allophones.

Voice-Voiceless

In the given corpus Robert appeared able to distinguish between the voiced and voiceless features. His use of "t" and "d" in /mtʊ du/ shows this contrast. Further material is needed to find out if this applies to fricatives.

Position

Robert uses five articulatory positions: bilabial as in /b/, labiodental as in /ʋ/, dental as in /ð/, alveolar as in /d/. He also uses a position that is in between the position for /tʃ/ and /ts/ as in /tṣ/.

No velar consonant in our language system was used although a velar position was used in /ɣ̊/ and /ʔ/ (glottal stop).

Obstruction

He uses four obstruction features. They are the fricative as in /s/, the liquid as in the dark /ɫ/, the nasal as in /m/, the plosive as in /b/.

It is at this stage we feel speech therapists should compare and contrast their language *system* with that of the dyslalic child. Having viewed the child's speech as a language system or code, we are bound to become interested in investigating what happens when the two respective linguistic systems come into contact with one another. Therefore the descriptive analysis must be complemented by a comparison. The following observations are the ones we consider to be the most interesting.

From work on the corpus under discussion it appears that Robert was minus ten of our phonemes, namely /k/, /g/, /ʃ/, /ʒ/, /tʃ/, /dʒ/, /ŋ/, /z/, /w/, /y/. This is taking into consideration that the corpus does not give an opportunity for all our phonemes to appear, /tʃ/ for example. The child does, however, use two phonemes which we do not have in our language system. They are /ɣ̊/ and /tṣ/. /ɣ̊/ is a voiceless pharyngeal sound and /tṣ/ is a voiceless sound made with the blade of the tongue against the teeth. He also makes more use of the glottal stop than we do. To help us with our further observations and to make it easier to contrast various features we divided the phones which resembled our phonemes into three headings – front, middle and back. These groups we divided into sub-groups of plosives, fricatives, nasals and semi-vowels.

FRONT	MIDDLE	BACK
p b	t d	K g
f v	ð θ	ʃ ʒ
s z	n	ŋ
w	y	h

This chart which – it should be emphasized – is only a rough guide, allows of a number of observations.

First, stress does not appear to influence any of the sounds. Second, taking each sound in turn, their incidence can be ascertained. /p/ in this corpus can only occur once and it is replaced by the glottal stop as in /tsoʔ/. /b/ is used in a one-to-one correspondence with ours and this could mean that /p/ and /b/ do not follow the same rules in Robert's system. However, the corpus is too small to draw any definite conclusions. /k/ and /g/ do not appear to be needed in his system. /d/ he uses as a free variant or interchangeably with /ð/ as in "the" and "de", or "then" and "den". (An example of a free variant in our language is the rolled and fricative *r*). It is possible that further investigation may show that the two sounds are allophones or members of the same phoneme and not the two separate phonemes we use. /d/ also corresponds to our /g/ which he does not appear to use, as in /doʔ/ "got". /t/ he seems to use in a one-to-one correspondence with our /t/. /f/ corresponds with /θ/ as in /fru/; the distinction between these two does not seem to be clear. /v/ is used only once and corresponds to our /w/, although one might expect this sound to correspond to /ð/ as /f/ corresponds to /θ/. The small corpus hampers us in drawing a definite conclusion. /ð/, as mentioned before, is used as a free variant of /d/. However, when these two sounds follow one another as in ænd /ðɛn/ Robert uses them according to our rules.

Sometimes he appears to try to make /ʃ/ and the result is a voiceless dental spirant.

He does not clearly distinguish /ʃ/ and /s/ as shown the first and last times he says "fish" – /fɪʔs, fɪ/.

He uses /m/ as a free variant of /n/ as in /ʋaʊm/ and /ʋaʊn/ though he uses the labio-dental nasal which is an allophone of /m/ in front of the labio-dental frictionless continuant, as we would use it in the word "comfort". This sound is, therefore, conditioned – it is under the influence of neighbouring or nearby phonetic features or elements. /ŋ/ does not appear in the corpus.

/h/ is a non-lingual dental spirant, that is, there is no tongue movement and it appears to be equivalent to the glottal stop as in /ʔoʊl/.

/tʂ/ may be an attempt to say /st/ in this context, the sound is midway between /ts/ and /tʃ/. It is not clear what he means by /tsoʔ ɪm/. The first supposition was that it was /st/ of "stop im", but it could just as easily be "got" or "chop". Unfortunately it does not occur often enough for conclusions to be drawn.

/ʔ/ is used as an all purpose plosive. It occurs as a free variant of /ɣ̊/ as in /fiʔ/ and /fiɣ̊/. He uses the glottal stop in between vowels as /biʔi/ and to correspond with our "h" as in /ʔoʊl/. Where it appears in front of a vowel as a strong vocalic onset it is not in contrast with another sound and is therefore non-distinctive. The glottal stop also appears in this corpus as a conditioned variant of the bilabial and alveolar position as in /deʔɪm/ and /tsoʔɪm/. That is, the glottal stop and /t/ or /p/ never occur in the same environment and, should they do so, the meaning of the word would be unchanged. An example of a conditioned variant in our language system is the clear "l" and the dark "l". It also appears that the glottal stop can occur in the same position and in place of a voiceless plosive as in /deʔ/. The glottal stop occurs far more often than in standard English. It is resorted to for more than emphasis.

/ɣ̊/ is used as an all purpose fricative. It is a back fricative and an unusual sound. A vowel always precedes it and it is in free variation with the glottal stop as in /fiɣ̊/, /fiʔ/ and /biɣ̊/, /biʔ/. In some places it is equivalent to our "g" as in /biɣ̊/.

Often we just do not know what the child is saying and then we are likely to jump to conclusions, giving our interpretation of a word which is quite likely to be different from what the child actually said. We should remember that "meaning is an integral part of language and hence cannot be eliminated from linguistic statements" (Jakobson, 1956).

In this corpus /ɣ̊/ corresponds with our /ʃ/ as in "fish", /t/ as in "got" and /z/ as in "was". This sound is not therefore a substitution as he has not the phonemes /ʃ/, /t/, /z/ to substitute. Communication theory has established that "only a limited number of signals can be used in any communicating system for speech since an infinite number would be impossible to remember and too cumbersome to be of service" (Pike, 1947). Can this sound really be a substitution with all that the word implies? We feel that /ʃ/, /t/, /z/ are redundant in Robert's language. "Redundancy is an essential ingredient of a communicative system, as flexible and broad in its coverage as language" (Pike, 1947).

From these observations we realize that Robert does not have difficulty in articulating phones – this is shown by his use of consonant clusters. His difficulty seems to lie in a lack of awareness of the phonological significance or importance of the English phonemic distinctions, which he treats as allophonic differences, as shown in his use of /d/ and /ð/. The phonemes which he has the most difficulty in discriminating are those that carry a low functional burden, for example /f/, /θ/, /m/, /n/.

All children begin their language development with coarse distinctions and progress step by step to finer discriminations. Robert has not progressed far enough. In systematizing his model he contrasts various features of the sounds, in patterns different from the conventional ones. He has organized the features of the language he has learned into his own language. In other words the limitations in Robert's speech are functional, not articulatory. Within his language there are "faults" only in that it differs from our own language and it is this aberrant linguistic system that must be rectified, not his so-called articulatory patterns. Therefore we must help Robert to develop linguistically by influencing him to reorganize the features he has already organized into his own language and to contrast features into our conventional patterns from his own unconventional ones.

The conclusions we draw as to the structure of his language must only be tentative as the corpus is so small. However, it would appear that there is a shift towards the middle position, that is, towards the middle or back of the oral cavity. This is shown in /f/ corresponding to /θ/. Also there is a tendency to weaken plosives as shown in /d/ to /ð/, /g/ to /ɣ̊/. There is not enough material for us to prove definitely how many phonemes there are in his linguistic system. It remains to be investigated among other things whether he employs /d/ and /ð/ as phonemes or allophones, whether he distinguishes between the voice-voiceless quality of /p/, /b/, and in what other environments he uses /ts/, if at all.

For this we shall need a larger corpus. We must have a larger number of phonemic analyses of the language of dyslalic children in order to prove incontrovertibly that our thesis, namely, that dyslalia is a language disorder, is a valid one.

REFERENCES

Harris, S. Z. (1951) *Methods in Structural Linguistics*, University of Chicago

Hockett, C. F. (1958) *A Course in Modern Linguistics*, New York, Macmillan

Pei, M. A., and Gaynor, F. (1954) *Dictionary of Linguistics*, London, Peter Owen

Jakobson, R., and Halle, M. (1956) *Fundamentals of Language*, The Hague, Mouton

Pike, K. (1947) *Phonemics*, Oxford University Press

17

P. A. E. GRADY, Nottingham

Towards a New Concept of Dyslalia

The aim of this chapter is to present further observations upon the disorder generally termed dyslalia and, by reference to the two preceding chapters, to indicate why it may be desirable to formulate a new concept of dyslalia.

In 1953 Macdonald Critchley delivered the Semon lecture and chose as his subject "Articulatory Defects in Aphasia". He said "throughout the literature upon speech disorders there is a regrettable tendency to confuse the terms 'language' and 'speech'". This tendency apparently persists today, even in the writings of speech therapists, and, although it is unimportant if the general public uses these words inter-changeably, it is fundamental to speech therapy that a distinction should be made between them.

Preliminary investigations of the nature of a patient's speech disorder should include procedures designed to facilitate a tentative diagnosis before treatment begins, in order to discover whether the patient's speech shows a defect of articulation or a defect in his language system. If a decision is made beforehand then treatment has a two-fold purpose. A manner of procedure may be specifically devised rather than applying a set formula, and it can teach the therapist, should her diagnosis be incorrect, how to approach similar disorders in the future. By regarding treatment as a means of confirming the tentative diagnosis it is hoped that magic will eventually be banished from speech therapy.

Although it is frequently postulated that speech therapy is not a form of symptomatic treatment, that is, that speech therapists do not simply correct mispronunciations, all too often treatment is started before a diagnosis has been made. The disappearance of a patient's speech disorder is not always positive proof of successful treatment. It is as well to remember that there has been little opportunity, so far, for speech therapists to include in their own programmes examinations of patients several years after discharge, and until numerous follow-up examinations are carried out it will remain unknown in what number of patients one symptom has been supplanted by another. A ten-year-old boy was recently re-referred to one of our clinics. Case notes showed that he had been treated for dyslalia at five years and that he had made a rapid improvement. In view of his subsequent difficulties in expressing himself fluently through speech it is interesting to note that one reason for treating him as an infant was because "speech has deteriorated since he started school when the pressure for correct speech became greater". At the present time this boy is reported to be unwilling to talk in school, he has a reading problem and an incipient stammer. He had a personal history of excessive dribbling and his tongue movements even now are clumsy. The boy seems to brace himself, giving the impression of a stammer, before he speaks. Both his parents and his teachers talk of some deterioration in speech little realizing how much effort the boy has to use to maintain the standard imposed by them – a demand that was unwittingly reinforced by speech therapy.

Treatment of a dyslalic child can so easily be called successful if the child gradually acquires the language system of his environment. The speech and language of these children should be re-examined from time to time in an attempt to find out if the label "dyslalic" was attached to their speech without reason and there should be a review of all the preliminary investigations carried out that led to the tentative diagnosis.

It is difficult to trace the origin of the word dyslalia to show how it came to be used in its present sense. Hippocrates and Aristotle both described several types of speech disorder – for example, speech in which the speaker was thought to substitute one sound for another, indistinct speech and speech characterized by omissions of speech sounds, but none of these was called dyslalia. In 1811 Johann Frank applied the word "dyslaliae" – the plural – to defects of articulation and other nineteenth-century writers followed suit. Dyslalia only means "to speak wrongly" and is, therefore, as vague a description as stomach-ache. It has a limited use for the purpose of indicating what is really wrong with the patient. Speech therapists, just as the doctor who examines a patient with stomach-ache, need more precise information before treatment can begin. A reappraisal of the definition is essential to prove whether it serves one of its uses, namely to indicate the nature of a patient's speech difficulty. The Terminology for Speech Pathology, recently published by the College of Speech Therapists, defined dyslalia as: "Defects of articulation, or slow development of articulatory patterns, including substitutions, distortions, omissions and transpositions of sounds of speech".

It seemed interesting to find out whether clinical experience with dyslalic patients supported the definition given by the College of Speech Therapists, bearing in mind Van Thal's presidential address at the 1952 Oxford Conference in which she warned members that

"The vexed question of terminology will never be settled till we have a more exact knowledge of the nature and cause of speech disorders. We must master semantics, and not believe in the magic of words, hoping that if we only prescribe a word to be used in given circumstances we shall have found the solution."

At this juncture it is pertinent to comment on the order of words in her phrase "nature and cause". As speech therapists, we wish to make a contribution to research into causes of speech disorders, but we should not search quite so diligently for diagnostic signs without first describing the nature of the patients' speech and language in terms that can be understood by workers in other specialties. However helpful it may seem for students of speech therapy to be given convenient labels for types of patients they meet during their first stages of clinical practice, there is nothing to be gained from attempting to fit patients into categories unless the *criteria* for establishing such categories, as well as the *purpose* of any classification, have been clearly stated. Speech therapists need to find out why each patient speaks as he does.

To say a patient has a defect of articulation means that he is unable to pronounce certain speech sounds. Defective articulation aptly describes dysarthric speech in which the patient is prevented from articulating all or some speech sounds according to the degree of inco-ordinated movements of his tongue, soft-palate, lips, etc. Robert, whose speech was analysed phonemically, was not handicapped in this way. Although his phonemes differ from those used by other members of his family and his speech includes the use of some non-English sounds he was not unable to articulate sounds. The phonemic differences that exist in various languages cannot be caused by individuals being unable to say certain sounds.

Before a patient is said to have "slow development of articulatory patterns" it would be helpful to know what is meant by articulatory patterns. Is it another way of saying the child is slow to imitate the speech and language of his social environment? If this is so, his failure to imitate would give rise to a speech disorder but would not be the disorder itself; cause is not the same as effect. It is unacceptable to say it depends on *how* the word "substitution" is used to say whether or not it describes Robert's speech. Substitution, in reference to speech, means that one phoneme is used instead of another one. The word "substitution" cannot be used if its meaning includes an implication that this is unconscious behaviour on the part of a child.

A series of transcriptions would show if phonemic differences are transient and haphazard, as for instance in slips of the tongue, and can rightly be described as mistakes. In Robert's case the application of such a test shows that this is not so. To think in terms of mistakes would influence the approach to treatment, reducing it to a form of speech correction and implying anticipation of a time when the child will rectify his own mistakes.

Before we accept it as axiomatic that a dyslalic child omits phonemes, it is necessary to prove that his language system once included the phonemes now thought to be missing. Certain patients with an acquired dysarthria may omit phonemes because they no longer possess the muscular ability to produce them, but a dyslalic child, as far as we know, has no similar disability. The study of Robert's language suggests that other dyslalic children may, on investigation, show the phonemic content of their language to be smaller than ours. One explanation of this would be that such children are unaware of the phonemic contrasts we make. Dyslalic children may find their own language adequate for their needs. If this assumption is correct then a moralistic judgement that dyslalic speech is wrong because it is different is not going to help treatment; it is more likely to hinder it.

It also becomes increasingly clear that we cannot say dyslalic speech is characterized by distortions of speech sounds. The term "distortion" may perhaps be reserved for some types of cleft-palate speech in which the listener finds it difficult to understand what a speaker with excessive nasality is saying. When referring to dyslalic speech it may be more accurate to say the patient "uses a different system of allophones". The so-called distortions can be represented by symbols, and once these are used, the listener is able to decide upon the phonemic features of the phones used by the speaker. Renfrew (1950) states "the judging of the point at which a sound is defective will always be a matter for subjective measurement." It is suggested that in dyslalic speech there is no necessity to make a subjective measurement. When we talk we use various allophones according to the environment of a particular phoneme. We may, if we wish, inter-change allophones and although the listener will notice something odd about our speech, the meaning will still be clear and conversation will not be impossible. When faced with the problem of unintelligible dyslalic speech our task, as speech therapists, should be to find out whether, for instance, /k/ is phonemically distinct from /t/ in a child's language as a means of translating what a child is saying. Hockett (1947) said:

> "The phonemes of a language, then are the elements which stand in contrast with each other in the phonological system of language.... It must be constantly remembered that a phoneme in a given language is defined only in terms of its differences from other phonemes in the same language."

If the wording of the authorized definition of dyslalia is correct, it would be possible for speech therapists to test a child's speech for the so-called faults already discussed. If dyslalia is a defect of articulation there should be no insuperable problems over devising a sound-test to be used as a preliminary aid to treatment. In such tests emphasis is laid on methods of eliciting a controlled response, but however carefully a test is prepared the response, often a single word, is of doubtful value. It is difficult to ensure that a child's response, in any test situation where speech is required, is a true mouth may be affected. On occasion the patient may exhibit contortions of the face in weeping and laughing which display a greater amount of emotion than he wishes to convey. The expression in the eyes can communicate the state of the patient's awareness of his environment.

Gesture

Gesture has three functions: to express emotion, to reinforce the meaning of the words uttered and to describe by other means than in words. As an instinctive physical reaction to internal and external stimuli a child uses gesture before he learns to speak. As he learns the use of language he makes gestures to reinforce his words. In naming an object he points to it, reaches out for it and becomes aquainted with the thing as he utters its name. Later he learns patterns of behaviour simultaneously with patterns of speech (such as waving "ta-ta!") and uses gesture as a means of expression when his words are inadequate (as in the familiar test to describe a spiral staircase). Gesture retains for most people its spontaneous emotional element, its reinforcing power and its descriptive features in communication.

The completely aphasic patient, if conscious of his surroundings, is responsive to the gestures of others and can make some response to his environment by the use of gesture himself. (The patient who hastily hides a dirty patch on her sheet is not entirely unresponsive to her surroundings. In contrast, the patient who is suffering from dementia is unaware of his surroundings and so unable to communicate with others.) Yet it must not always be assumed that the aphasic patient's gesture means what it seems to mean. For instance, a patient nods his head, apparently in assent. This is a positive, a friendly gesture, a response to a voice, but it cannot be taken for granted that the patient has understood or is agreeing to what has been said. The clue of apparent consent may lead up a blind alley! The negative shake of the head indicates refusal and withdrawal but not necessarily a direct "no" in answer to a question. The use of a meaningful nod or shake of the head in answer to questions was used by Douglas Ritchie (1960) and his wife as a means of communication, but was very tedious and gave rise to misunderstandings at times.

An aphasic patient's gestures may indicate his state of mind – excitement, pleasure, frustration, anger – but do not always elucidate the ideas he is seeking to express. Some patients are ingenious in their use of gesture in an attempt to convey meaning but in most cases their sign language is limited, and an arm pointing in one direction may mean "far away", "at home", "yesterday", "years ago", or a person who is not present, on different occasions or even in the same conversation.

There is a fundamental difference between the child's gesture which he is associating with the object that he is learning to name and so to apprehend and the aphasic concentrating his effort within himself to find the word which is already his but which cannot be uttered. To such an adult it is distracting to attempt to perform action and speech together, as in naming a letter at the moment of writing it. For him it is "one thing at a time". Though an attempt must be made to re-open all paths of communication through speech, reading and writing, they cannot all be traversed simultaneously.

For other aphasic patients the use of canalized patterns of movement accompanied by sounds are helpful in evoking words. The child learning to speak may associate certain gestures with the words "ta" and "bye-bye"; similarly the aphasic may use hand movements in "up", "down", "come", "go" and so on, to reinforce his verbal expression. This is a process of learning and in my experience was found to be helpful for a Polish woman who had to relearn English after her stroke, and also for a young woman who, as the result of severe cerebral damage, reverted to childish habits of behaviour and only gradually learned to walk and to talk again.

At a conference on "Stroke Rehabilitation" it was suggested by a speaker that aphasic patients should be taught a sign language by means of which they could communicate. In my opinion, if formalized gestures (as opposed to spontaneous ones) are taught, the patient should always make an attempt to say the word with the gesture. This may then be a means to the end of evoking speech. But the time spent in teaching a systematized and comprehensive form of gesture language to an adult aphasic could surely be more profitably occupied in attempting to re-awaken his former use of spoken and written language.

If a patient can use signs intelligibly he will use them spontaneously when words fail him, and he need not be taught. The use of gesture should not be inhibited. Signs, drawing and writing can all be used to aid communication and to help to reawaken the power of speech.

Articulation

The clues that might be followed in observing the articulatory disturbances in aphasia are a subject for study which cannot be considered in any detail here.

Disorders of articulation may occur separately or in combination with disorders of language. A patient may be suffering from dysarthria and dyspraxia in addition to being dysphasic and a close observation of the articulation will give a clue as to whether he has a disorder of articulation as well as a disturbance of the higher and more complex function of language. The disordered speech patterns of the dysarthric patient are predictable and more or less consistent in their form though they deteriorate as the patient becomes fatigued. The articulatory errors of a patient who is suffering from dysphasia are unpredictable and inconsistent. Mere fragments of a word may be uttered, or consonant combinations may be simplified, or feeble attempts at speech may produce slurred articulation. Extra effort in speaking may cause sound distortions in executive dysphasia, and lack of perception may account for the errors when there is a receptive loss. The physical condition of the patient, especially when he is fatigued, will influence his manner of speaking. Enunciation deteriorates if the intellect is impaired, and speech may degenerate to earlier patterns of movement and sounds. The quiet reiterative babbling of some aphasic patients shows signs of this degeneration.

Macdonald Critchley (1953, p. 8) points out that "in the dilapidated speech of aphasics it is often easy to pick up audible traces of a regional or provincial accent", and that "there is evidence that after the onset of an aphasia, dialect may become exaggerated or perhaps merely re-emerge".

Language

No word used by an aphasic patient, however irrational it may seem in its context, is produced without a cause, or chain of causes. If we question why did he say that (what does it signify?), we may be led to a fuller understanding of the functioning of the patient's mind.

The type of language disorder found in amnesic aphasia is similar to that from which we all suffer at times. The word-finding difficulty is noticeable when we are tired, lacking in attention or over-anxious. We may say "What-you-m'-call-it" or "thing-a-m'-jig" or any one of a number of such "words" in place of the name. The rhythm and ring of these substitutions and the use of a falling intonation indicates satisfaction with the substitute – "It's on the what's-it in the kitchen." If we really seek the word there is a tendency to use a rising intonation and answer the query. "It's on the what-you-call-it? . . . the dresser in the kitchen."

The aphasic is seeking a word which he has not lost entirely but he cannot find the particular "pigeon-hole" (so to speak) in which the word is located and he has to search the area round about. (A patient named a petrol driven bicycle as "Oh, over the crest and away".)

The aphasic who has difficulty in formulating his thoughts is suffering from a lack of central control. Fragments of sentences are uttered and "jumping-off" phrases keep obtruding themselves meaninglessly. This also occurs with so-called "normal" speakers: the aphasic does it to excess. Many people intersperse their sentences with "you sees" and "you knows", and some rapid, excitable speakers clutter, omit words and jump ahead in their speech. Normally a speaker can control this by "taking thought", but when control is disorganized in aphasia disordered sentences emerge. (A patient was to write a sentence containing the word WOOD. He wrote, "Wooden by others you can name." I asked, "What does it mean?" He replied, "Not a great to people like you." "What does it mean to you?" "Rather a lot. The window are made up in special woods." "What others can you name?" "This is rather an awkward one for me this is. Wooden that's right and understood as hardwood, number 5, and wood which would be the usual is number 7." The man was a builder.

Words have for each of us a network of associations, some of universal significance, others of purely personal meaning. These associations refer to all aspects of the word, auditory, visual and kinaesthetic, linked with personal experiences. For the aphasic these become tangled, disconnected or so closely held that thought cannot be free to use other paths.

Association of ideas can be used to help an aphasic to recall words. For example, a patient was able to repeat the following words, after a week, when the linking ideas were given. "House, door, key, open, window, summer, garden, flowers." The danger of giving words that are too closely linked is that the patient may perseverate like a gramophone needle stuck in a groove.

The association may work on a subliminal level and the link be difficult to find. As an example of the normal functioning of the subconscious mind let me illustrate. The noise made by the engine of my car made me say to myself, "It's roaring like a young lion." A few minutes later, while consciously thinking of other things, I found myself singing, "Shall want no manner of thing that is good. . . ." The clue, which took some finding was, "The young lions do lack and suffer hunger, but they that seek the Lord . . ."

A patient was trying to describe the story of the Wounded Crow as seen in the View Master, and some time later came out unexpectedly with the word "taxidermist". In the photograph the crow does look as if it has been stuffed!

Rhythm and fluency

There are two types of hesitation shown by aphasics which closely follow the symptoms of stammering, the reiteration of sounds and the complete blocking of speech. Macdonald Critchley (1953, p. 14) suggests that there may be a link between stammering and aphasia, and that "stammering . . . may represent a disorder in the faculty of language". It is true that some aphasic patients present us with clues that may help us to relieve their "stammer". One such woman, suffering from executive aphasia and complete blockage of speech, wrote, "I count myself worn. My throat my tightness. I hope the beath" (I hold the breath).

Russell Brain (1951) wrote

> "The aphasic patient requires to be taught on lines similar to those used in teaching a backward child. The various vowel and consonant sounds must be taught separately, the patient being directed to watch the movements of the teacher's lips and tone . . ."

and so on. I submit that this is true only for a limited number of patients, those who, because of the extent of the cerebral damage, have become as "backward children."

Language is not lost in aphasia but its functions are disturbed and the faculty must be re-established by the use of words in meaningful situations. Methods of helping individuals must vary and while every attempt is made to reawaken the memories of the sight, sound and kinaesthetic sensations of spoken and written language, communication can be more quickly established by using words in context.

Each aphasic patient is wandering in his own particular maze. We must follow with him the clues he offers and so help to guide him on his way back to normality.

REFERENCES

Lindsey Batten, Stroke Rehabilitation Conference, London, June 22, 1961
Concise Oxford Dictionary
Terminology for Speech Pathology, College of Speech Therapists (1959)
Ritchie, Douglas (1960) *Stroke*, London, Faber and Faber
Critchley, Macdonald "Articulatory Defects in Aphasia", The Semon Lecture, Reprinted in *Speech*, April 1953, p. 8
Brain, W. Russell (1951) *Diseases of the Nervous System*, Oxford University Press, p. 105

19

D. B. FITCH, London

The Assessment of Defective Speech in an Adult

The child patient is generally referred to the speech therapy department because of speech symptoms that reveal some deficiency. Speech has failed to develop normally and some lack in the patient's physical, intellectual or emotional equipment has become apparent. Diagnosis of the underlying condition is of paramount importance to the child's future development and examination of the speech and language behaviour is part of the diagnostic procedure.

The adult patient more frequently comes to the speech therapist as the result of a change of state concerning his physical or psychological condition. The pathology of the former may be stated by the physician or surgeon while the speech therapist assesses the abnormalities of the patient's speech and accompanying behaviour. She analyses the existing speech pattern and compares it with the pre-morbid pattern which she may know or deduce from the level of speech demanded by the patient's environment and profession, and observation of the patient's reaction to his disability; information from himself and his family complete the picture. The speech assessment must be based upon full comprehension of the factors that have brought about the change whether physical or psychological and it is carried out with a view to establishing a treatment-principle.

In other cases the speech disorder is not the result of a change of the patient's condition but an increasing discrepancy between what is demanded of the patient and what he can achieve. This is usually brought about by environmental changes, marriage, promotion or by the increasing age and responsibility of the patient which render previous speech habits unsuitable. In this group may be encountered patients with vocal disorders, some stammerers and patients with defective articulation, notably of "r" and "s". The increased discrepancy between demand and performance causes the person discomfort or distress and prompts him to seek help. The patient is not necessarily aware of what he is doing but he is aware that the result is not what he wishes to achieve. In these cases the therapist and patient are evaluating the speech performance, not against a previous normal standard, but against a possible future one. The discrepancy revealed in the assessment is not between what he was and what he is, but between what he is and what he wishes to be.

Assessing speech that is unquestionably defective must comprehend:

1. Identification of sounds produced, conventional or otherwise.
2. Observation of the state of the organs concerned with the production of sound and their movement and coordination.
3. Ascertainment of the patient's ability to hear, perceive and produce sounds other than those he now utters.
4. Ascertainment of the patient's ability to experience kinaesthetic and tactile sensations other than those he now experiences.
5. Investigation of the patient's attitude towards his speech.
6. Investigation of the amount of insight he has into his condition.

It must be emphasized that in assessing the defective speech of an adult the therapist is concerned as much with attitudes as with abilities. The patient has developed a means of communication that has been adequate and has become inadequate. His attitudes and abilities together have been responsible for the extent of his success and adjustment in the past and will be responsible for his success and adjustment in the future. The inter-relationship of the patient's attitudes and abilities built up over many years may make it difficult for the therapist to establish what is the main factor in the speech disturbance. She must make every effort to do so because her treatment directive depends upon the accuracy of the assessment.

The patient who presents real problems of assessment is the adult clutterer. The patient usually comes to the speech clinic, not as the result of a recently acquired disorder, nor of any discomfort or distress of his own about his speech performance, but because other people find him difficult to understand and think it necessary that he should improve. The nature of the speech disturbance, overhasty and inaccurate utterance, is such that the layman considers it could easily be corrected if the patient would take more care or make more effort. It is not realized that the patient is incapable of these measures because he is essentially unsure of his own speech performance and the effect of this upon others.

It is not the purpose of this paper to consider in general the behaviour and problems of the clutterer. There is considerable reference to these patients in the literature of speech pathology and particularly in the admirable articles by Godfrey E. Arnold, "Studies in Tachyphemia" published in *Logos* (1960).

It is proposed to consider one such patient with reference to the problems posed in the attempt to assess his abilities and performance and find a treatment directive from this assessment.

The patient, eighteen years of age, was referred to the speech therapist from the E.N.T. department. The terms of referral stated that there was no physical abnormality but that the patient spoke fast and inaccurately and people could not understand him. A subsequent report from the Neurological Department stated that there were no abnormal signs in the nervous system. It was considered by both the neurologist and the otolaryngologist that the patient was of above average intelligence and should benefit from speech therapy. This patient then became solely the concern of the speech therapist and the importance of the speech assessment was accordingly emphasized. Recordings of the patient's speech when played to other therapists produced widely different opinions all of which proved to be off the mark. They considered it to be: (1) dysarthria – this was discounted because of the absence of abnormal signs in the nervous system; (2) dyspraxia – this seemed possible but not sufficiently comprehensive; (3) dyslalia associated with poor mentality – this was disproved by the patient's intellectual attainments and pursuits; (4) poor grade speech – this was discounted because it was difficult to see why a patient coming from an environment of superior speakers should not approximate to his speech environment if he had the ability. In this patient's environment the quality of his speech must be considered defective. It was then realized that attempts to name the condition were not helpful in that they were based on insufficient examination and did not give rise to a treatment principle. The therapist considered that the descriptive term of Cluttering was the most helpful designation, but it was only upon reading Dr Arnold's articles at a later date that she was confirmed in this opinion (1960).

Case history

Premature baby – seven months. Mother had eclampsia during pregnancy. The infant was bottle fed. The patient's parents were both well educated and well spoken. There was no record of defective speech on either side of the family. Sent to day nursery every day from 8 a.m.–6 p.m. throughout infancy. The development of speech was late. Mother was uncertain as to the actual time of starting but said that he could read before he was able to speak sentences. She attributed the late speech and early reading to his time in the day nursery. The patient read fluently when he started school at five years. Later he went to a grammar school and did particularly well in mathematics but dropped Latin and French early. He had pronounced difficulty with spelling and was given special tuition. His spelling is still very erratic and unusual, and he writes quickly with repetition and elision of words and mistakes crossed out or left unrecognized. He had a routine hearing test at school and was declared normal. It was intended that he should go to university, but at sixteen years he was offered a job as an estimator at a paint factory. This promised to be interesting and had good prospects and the patient was adamant in choosing to accept it. The firm in question considered him to be brilliant at mathematics and generally able, but became concerned about his speech as it produced an adverse effect on others and occasionally prevented them from understanding him. It was in response to suggestions from the firm that the patient eventually came for treatment.

During his school years the patient's speech had always been fast and difficult to understand. His parents both considered that "the trouble was he spoke too fast, we used to tell him not to". They requested the removal of his tonsils and adenoids at seven years because of "a slight thickness in his speech" but there was no improvement. The patient at school was very good at rugby and even better at chess. He is now a county standard chess player.

Laterality

Started with preference for the left hand. Became right-handed at school. Mother was also left-handed and changed to right.

Appearance

The patient gave the impression of slight clumsiness in his general gait and in the performance of fine movements. His face was inexpressive in that his cheeks and upper lip seemed to lack mobility. He tended to look down or away from the speaker, was uncommunicative and appeared slightly resentful of the interest he was arousing. He displayed little interest in the original speech investigation and none at all in the general activity of the clinic. He would sit down in the out-patient department and read with absorption until called in, never looking up nor speaking to anyone. His choice of reading matter was generally concerned with chess or mathematical problems.

Speech

The first and general impression was that the speech was too fast, uncoordinated, variable and monotonous. There was a pronounced labial rhotacism and equally pronounced sigmatism varying from palatal to lateral. The lack of clarity was otherwise not related to the defective production of specific phonemes but to the extreme variability of the phonemic structure.

Illustrations of speech fluctuation

"Fly" was pronounced with a labial plosive initially [plaɪ] and with a labial fricative initially [Φlaɪ] in the same sentence. [p] was pronounced as a bi-labial plosive initially and medially in "puppy" and finally in "hope" but as a bi-labial fricative in "proper". The assimilation was not consistent because [p] was given correct labial plosion in "premonition" pronounced [primənitn] "premoniton". "th" [θ] was pronounced [f] in "thunder" and "thousand", [d] in "this". "s" in addition to the usual palatal substitution was example of how he normally speaks. The speech therapist faces the same problem met by any investigator when trying to obtain a sample of spontaneous speech – the subject either tries too hard or is overawed by the situation. Pike (1947) drew attention to this when he wrote, "In some types of speaking, especially in precise or school-room speech, phonemic contrasts are present which do not exist in normal speech." It is quite possible, therefore, to obtain varying results depending on the method of assessment used with dyslalic children. For example, Robert uses a glottal stop phonemically yet in routine tests this would be counted as zero.

Van Riper's (1959) statement that "we must discover the articulatory errors which make his speech unacceptable" suggests that a speech therapist's judgement is not only moralistic but based on aesthetic standards of correctness. If they are, the sound tests devised may well mark the child's "errors" by ticks and crosses or the addition and subtraction of points. There is great difficulty in obtaining a norm in order that a test result may be compared and contrasted with such a norm to make it possible for the score to be expressed either as a speech age or as a percentage. Scores are not entirely valueless if a sound-test is standardized but it is necessary to define the factor that is being tested. The multiplicity of intelligence tests shows there is no universally acceptable definition of intelligence; each test shows various aspects of intelligence.

Epstein (1960) pointed out "The term 'articulation testing' is therefore misleading as one does not test articulatory motor ability but purely central linguistic ability, namely the expressive unit of language". If an utterance is taken as the expressive unit, then the study of dyslalic speech should not be made upon a unit smaller than a single utterance, although this may, in some instances, consist of one syllable. Speech therapists learn to translate what a dyslalic patient is saying and find they take into account not only phonemic differences but make use of the child's stress, pitch and intonation. By approaching the problem of unintelligibility holistically they find a key to the code. Shames (1960) in a paper to members of the 1959 International Congress said that

> "The concept of speech intelligibility can so easily be fractionalized and be made to seem simpler than it really is by virtue

of our present crude methods of measurement. Intelligibility is a concept of language and its measurement, if it is to be valid, will have to account for the language factor."

There is increasing evidence to encourage a profound change in our attitude towards dyslalic patients. We should no longer look on these children as speech defectives, but as patients exhibiting signs of language disorder. We should continue to examine the system each child uses instead of compiling a list of faults and start treatment only when we have carried out more detailed examinations so that treatment is individual to the patient and verifies the diagnosis of his linguistic system.

The writers wish to thank Dr R. G. Sprenger for affording them the opportunity to carry out this work; Mr J. L. Trim and Mr W. Haas for their guidance in the preparation of these three papers and especially Dr Leopold Stein for his generous assistance and encouragement.

REFERENCES

Critchley, Macdonald (1953) *Speech* **XVII**, No. 1, April

Epstein, A. G. (1960) "Phonemic Testing", *J. South African Logopedic Society*, December

Frank, Johann (1811) *Praxeos Medicae Universae Precepta*, Leipzig

Hockett, Charles (1947) *A Course in Modern Linguistics*, New York, Macmillan

Pike, K. (1947) *Phonemics*, Oxford University Press

Renfrew, Catherine (1950) "A Measurement of Attainment in Articulation", *Speech* **XIV**, No. 2

Shames, G. H., and Fisher, J. (1960) "The Relationship of Types of Articulation Errors to Intelligibility of Speech", *Speech Pathology and Therapy* **III**, No. 1, April

Van Riper, Charles (1959) *Voice and Articulation*, London, Pitman

Van Thal, Joan (1952) Summary of President's Opening Address, Report of the Conference on Speech Therapy

18

JOYCE L. WILKINS, Nottingham

Clues in Aphasia

When Theseus entered the labyrinth to slay the Minotaur Ariadne gave him a clew of thread so that he might find his way out again.

The study of human speech and particularly that of the disturbed and disintegrated condition known as aphasia leads us into a labyrinth, a maze wherein we may easily become hopelessly lost.

While the neurologists and the neurosurgeons are surveying this area of human behaviour and making a map which may eventually be a complete guide to aphasia, it is the task of the speech therapist wandering in the maze to follow the clues offered by aphasic patients in order to effect the release of "the indwelling word that cannot be uttered" (Batten, 1961).

Aphasia is a disturbance of the function of language in which the perception and expression of the spoken and written word has been lost or impaired. We are concerned here with acquired aphasia.

A clue is a "fact or principle that serves as a guide, or suggests a line of inquiry in any problem, investigation or study" (*Concise Oxford Dictionary*). Spelt CLEW (which is derived from the same word) it is a ball of thread such as that which lead Theseus out of the maze. When we are "clueless" we are "without a clew!" Therefore it is proposed to follow some clues in aphasia which, when we are wandering in the labyrinth, may lead us to the centre of the individual patient's problem.

The problem is the breakdown of the ability to communicate through language. The patient has lost skills that he had acquired and on which he had come to rely, the ability to understand and to use words, and in particular spoken words, that is, speech.

Speech (according to the definition accepted by the College of Speech Therapists in 1959) "is the audible expression of language consisting of organized patterns of articulation". The term therefore embraces the whole audible act of speaking, the voice, the articulation, language and (in the organized patterns) rhythm and fluency. But there are also visible aspects of speaking that we must consider, namely: facial expression and gesture. Communication through the written word and pictures depends on the ability to use and interpret graphic symbols, lines and colour, and abstract their significance. The functions of both spoken and written language may be disturbed in aphasia, though some channels of communication may be left open.

Here we will consider particularly communication through speech. This depends on the voice, including pitch, volume, tone and the variety of intonation or speech melody, gesture, including facial expression and bodily movements, articulation, the patterns of movement and the speed of utterance, the words used in their context, and the rhythm and stress with which they are uttered. All these contribute to the expression of thought. The interpretation depends on the perception and understanding of the hearer. The first three – voice, gesture and articulation – are based on inherent abilities which are later canalized into conforming linguistic patterns, the latter – words in their contexts – are acquired symbols.

The first clue to follow then is: in spite of the loss of the use of the acquired symbols, is communication still possible through earlier modes of behaviour? If so, can these channels be used to help re-establish fuller communication?

Voice

The voice of the patient who has suffered a cerebral catastrophe will be affected at least temporarily if not permanently. A stroke strikes the whole person and his voice suffers in the shock. Complete aphonia may be the result of the neurological condition or the result of shock and acute fear. In the latter case the voice can be freed when anxiety is relieved and the muscular tension released. An indication that voice is still possible is the ability to cough and to laugh. If this ability has remained the patient can be encouraged in the belief that he can produce voice and treatment may be directed to that end.

For some the aphonia may be a form of psychological withdrawal, the result of a need for a time of silence, and should be respected as such. Dr Stein, in a personal communication, said:

> "Silence is also a form of communication. The need for silence varies. The aphasic's reaction to his own enforced silence may be an important clue to treatment. Perhaps in certain cases we should not be too eager to 'make' him speak."

Much can be learned of the patient's state of mind as well as of his physical condition by listening to his voice, its volume, pitch, and tone as well as to the intonation used. The unnaturally high-pitched voice is indicative of excitement, nervous strain or excessive effort and is associated with shallow, clavicular breathing. The trembling voice and "childish pipe" may be a sign of senile degeneration; the nasal escape an indication of loss of muscular tone; strident tones and loss of volume and power all give clues to the patient's physical condition and psychological state.

The intonation may convey more than is implied by the halting words spoken. As with a small child learning to read, the tune is not related to the words but to the effort involved in speaking and to a request for assurance. There is the diffident underlying "is that right?" speech melody, the hopelessly negative and frustrated "I can't" tune, and the conciliatory "I am trying, don't be cross" intonation. These may not be suitable to the words and the situation in which they are spoken but they may be an indication of the underlying conflict in the mind of the patient.

The aphasic patient, like the child before he has learned to use words, can yet appreciate the tones of voice of those who speak to him, and respond to them. (Only one who has completely lost contact with reality does not respond, and his own confused utterance is an indication of his state.) When an aphasic patient is using fluent jargon or a reiterative phrase there is often an underlying meaning in his intonation, indicating an inner awareness and desire to communicate though the words may be "meaningless". Obviously in short utterances such as "No! no! no!" when the patient really means "Yes! yes! yes!" the speech melody is of no help, but on many occasions tone and tune can convey the meaning.

Facial expression can be a help in conveying meaning, but muscular response may be slow and in hemiplegia the movements of the replaced by [θ] in "seeking the secret of success", elided after the [k] in "ecstasy", replaced by [ʃ] in "anxious". [g] was articulated correctly in the word "gome" which was the patient's pronunciation of "gnome". It was replaced by [b] in "agreeable" and "disgruntled" and by [d] in "green". [k] was correct in "care" and in "curiosity". It was replaced by a lateral fricative in "club" but was correctly pronounced in "Clementine". It was replaced by a labial fricative in "accrue" and by [ks] in "acquisition".

In view of the numerous instances of elision and assimilation in the speech the listening ability was explored. The patient could not at first distinguish between "s" or "sh", and "f" and "th" and "s" in isolation. He identified a gross lateral fricative and palatal fricative in isolation as being different from "s" but did not pick them out when uttered less strongly or prominently in words. [r], [l] and [j] could not at first be distinguished consistently from each other in isolation. The patient showed poor ability to identify sounds in nonsense words.

These observations support the contention that the clutterer listens for meanings, not sounds. This was also supported by the patient's attitude to his own recorded speech. He understood himself perfectly and did not consider his speech at all defective. When recordings of his speech were played back several weeks later the result was the same, as the patient remembered what he had said and understood himself.

During any period of listening and sound imitation the patient appeared distressed and strained. He would screw up his eyes or stare into space. Nonsense syllables were imitated in a staccato fashion with apparent attempts to retain the auditory pattern by effort.

The patient scored better on identifying words that were mispronounced, e.g. epilesy for epilepsy, acclimize for acclimatize, solomonization for solemnization. He could not identify the exact error in epilepsy but could say the word correctly himself, acclimatize he could not repeat correctly, saying acclimanize, and solemnization he could recognize as mis-pronounced yet not distinguish the error nor say the word correctly himself.

He would not repeat "ta ta ta" "ta ta ta" quickly and lightly nor vary the stress, saying he did not like the combination of sounds. "Ka ka ka" he was induced to try with different rhythms, but found this difficult. "Ta ka ta ka" was very difficult but "pa ta pa ta" and "pa ta pa" were performed with comparative ease.

Any pattern of sound, however simple, caused difficulties of imitation, as did tapping and clapping of rhythms and following any simple tune.

Singing

He would attempt to sing something he had often heard but rendered it in a distorted fashion. The notes were unduly prolonged and produced in a throaty constricted manner. It seems very likely that this was associated with poor ability to perceive the pitch changes. He could not imitate a simple cadence and could only distinguish between notes of very different pitch. The singing ability of the rest of the family is good and a maternal uncle is a professional singer.

Ability to imitate a simple intonation pattern was very poor and together with singing produced very effortful and painful grimaces and eye screwing.

Tongue movements

The tongue could be protruded, moved laterally and elevated and the sides rolled up but there was little ability to point the tip. There was little response when the sides and tip were scratched with a spatula. The tongue seemed to be broad and large and it appeared to move without delicacy although the movements intended were adequately controlled. The palate appeared to elevate well.

During the assessment and subsequent treatment the patient was cooperative and diligent but showed a lack of ease and certainty. At any point of failure or breakdown in his ability to produce or reproduce sounds he showed a mild catastrophic reaction. The effect produced was of a scatter of impressions and a desperate attempt to hold them together.

The dominating fact emerging from the attempt at assessment is the patient's lack of ability to monitor his speech.

The following indications for treatment arise:

1. To arouse interest in the sounds of speech.
2. To improve auditory attention and memory for sound and for tune and rhythm.

3. To encourage the patient to rely more on auditory information and less on visual.

4. To encourage him to understand and appreciate the effect of speech upon other people.

5. To maintain his cooperation throughout the entire procedure by giving him specific tasks wherever possible.

6. To draw his attention to the sounds which are most consistently deviate and mispronounced – "r" and "s" – and to bring these nearer to their accepted phoneme, thereby to reduce the amount of assimilation in contiguous sounds.

I wish to thank Mr V. Hammond, F.R.C.S., for his original referral and subsequent interest in the patient and Miss Prudence Oliver, L.C.S.T., for her help in assessment and treatment.

REFERENCES

Arnold, G. E. (1960) "Studies in Tachyphemia (I)", *Logos* **3**, No. 1, April

Arnold, G. E. (1960) "Studies in Tachyphemia (III)", *Logos* **3**, No. 2, October

20

LYN P. PARKER, Newcastle

A Critical Investigation into the Problem of Dysarthria

In an article which appeared in the *Listener* in August, 1960, entitled "Science is Social", John Ziman said

> "the act of writing up one's results is not a tiresome chore and a distraction from 'real' research, it is a highly creative activity, for we do not always know exactly what we have discovered until we set it down on paper for others to read".

My original purpose then was to ascertain what I have gathered from what others have discovered regarding the diagnostic entity known as dysarthria, in an attempt to clarify what is meant by the term dysarthria and to delineate its place in the whole field of disturbance of speech and language. The main points of a few writers shall be presented in the hope that this may stimulate discussion and thought and the desire to delve deeper into the problem of dysarthria.

It is intended to view critically that which has been written and to try to integrate this material, so that we may know what it is that we know, and what it is that we think we know. It is well to remember that most writers will have already appreciated the arguments against their writings and have presented their theories for the purpose of having them corroborated or disproved, and they should, therefore, be viewed in a constructive manner.

How can we be sure of basic facts in a field of such complexity as language, where the integration of such functions as are believed to be fundamental is such that none can be separated one from the other? Only a careful analysis and interpretation of what has already been written and a critical scrutiny of our own observations and statements will provide this. Upon these we may then base further deliberations conducive to purposive research in our endeavour to find out whether what has been assumed to be true is true.

Since the definition of dysarthria presupposes that of the widest concept of articulation it seems advisable before investigating the problem of dysarthria to know what is meant by articulation. It is generally agreed that articulation is the process of producing the sounds used in speech by means of movements of the lips, jaw, tongue and palatopharyngeal mechanism in coordination with respiration and phonation. Yet most authorities on dysarthria do not go further than what descriptive phonetics purports to state regarding the mechanics involved. What seems to be needed is to make at least assumptions as to how this ability comes about. We over-simplify by taking articulation away from the rest of the process of communicative speech and define it too narrowly as a motor function. What makes matters worse is that the classifier often remains oblivious of the purpose of his grouping.

Penfield says, "Articulation depends upon the employment of special motor areas in the cortex of either hemisphere" (1958), and shows that cortical control of articulatory movements and vocalization is located between the two principal areas for ideational speech, one posterior and one anterior, that is, in the posterior temporal and posterior-inferior parietal regions and a small area in the posterior part of the third frontal convolution. The streams of neurone impulses that produce voluntary movements arise in the circuits of integration in the brain stem – the centrencephalic system. "These impulses", he says, "flow out to these cortical motor areas and from there down to the muscles of mouth and throat and diaphragm."

Such neuro-anatomical and neurophysiological facts confirmed by scientific experiments and observations can readily be accepted by us, and it is of course left to us to utilize them in our endeavour to gain some insight into the dynamism operative on the various levels of spoken language.

Goldstein (1954) does not define articulation but he clearly regards it as a complex function, saying:

cases in comparison with the normal speech of normal people. In Group 4 (slowly developing speech) there were children whose speech was normal for their mental age. They were not, however, included in Group 5 (normal speech) as their speech fell below the standard of the speech of children of a similar chronological age. Children in Group 5 were for the most part children with either a good speech ability, a favourable speech environment or both.

The speech therapist saw every child in the centre and selected her cases. The children were reviewed at six to twelve monthly intervals, in some instances more frequently, and were placed in the following groups:

(*a*) Those in need of speech therapy.

(*b*) Those unable at the time of review to benefit from treatment.

(*c*) Those needing treatment for a specific aspect of speech (e.g. vocabulary building).

(*d*) Those needing help only on general lines, of a kind suited to the needs of the "backward" child.

It was then possible to draw up a scheme which was individually suited to the needs of the centre under survey and the children in any class could be grouped according to their special needs. In these centres there are many children whose speech disorder is based on a neurological condition and these should be under the care of the speech therapist who is aware of the factors at work in such conditions as, for instance, dysarthria.

A loving and permissive atmosphere, with time for nursery play and work and the chance to chatter and make noise freely – these, within a secure background of order and periods of rest and quiet, are best for the less mature and the younger children. In speech they achieve more than those who have only formal speech training, who are handled formally and expected to sit still, to be quiet and so on. Our observations extending over a period of years tally with those of others in this field and have been verified experimentally. Being noisy, babbling, learning words for daily use and later learning simple phrases are all part of the training needed. A vocabulary of use and interest to the child with frequent repetitions can be gradually introduced by the speech therapist. Speech has to be learnt in every lesson and daily activity, including the lessons in music, dancing and acting. Wherever commands are given, listening power and comprehension are being trained. Thus while speech training is needed, the acquisition of speech should never be isolated from daily life but constantly be introduced as a pleasant and social activity.

In assessing the children's speech I see it as a social and emotional function and ask myself, "Is the child 'focused' adequately in his relationships with people? Does he use objects meaningfully for their correct purpose and for play? Is he withdrawn or astray? Does he use objects for stereotyped repetitive motions? Does he converse only if questioned? Will he speak only when told to repeat after someone?" In such cases speech is produced, if it is at all possible, by helping the child to make better contact with people. In cases where the behaviour is related to a very low I.Q. or brain damage rather than to psychosis, the achievement of a small amount of speech on a realistic level is valuable.

The social aspect of speech is especially important for these children since they have such a limited contact with the world that they cannot comprehend well, have few means of occupying leisure and will in later life be in the care of strangers.

To aid assessment and diagnosis children are observed in their classrooms and given both formal and informal interviews. Teachers and social workers are consulted in order to decide whether the deviations from normal speech are in keeping with the child's intellectual and emotional capacity or whether treatment is advisable. Here the following criteria may be of use: (1) The presence of speech defects of moderate to severe degree (deviations from the normal) where mental age, general ability and organic state suggest that an improvement in the child's speech can be expected. It is as well to judge the child by observation and report rather than to rely only on the results of intelligence tests. Performance on tests may be affected by poor speech. The intelligence quotient is not the only criterion in prognosis. The desire to please and to communicate lead some very "dull-seeming" children to be more self-active and to persevere. Some children seem to have a poorer specific ability for speech than for other activities. Some, who receive insufficient home teaching and stimulation to speak may need only periodic speech therapy supplemented by advice to parents and teachers. Some children's characteristics overlap with those of the next category.

(2) The presence of speech disorders of moderate to severe degree due to conditions other than lack of intellect alone, such as dysarthria, dysphasia, articulatory dyspraxia and so on. Severe cases of disorders such as dysphonia and marked dysarthria respond less well than cases of disorders of language and articulation where there is a possible basis of dysphasia and allied conditions. This should be borne in mind when deciding upon the advisability of treatment but it may be wise to give such cases a trial. The stammering of mongols may be difficult to treat, perhaps because the nature of this type of stammering is not clear enough to conduce to any rational therapeutic approach.

(3) The presence of some physical abnormality or handicap which affects the speech. For instance, malformation of tongue or jaws, slight hearing loss and so on, to which these children cannot adapt (though adaptation is possible).

(4) The ability (after several trials if need be) to repeat sounds or words correctly.

(5) The absence of the wish to vocalize or speak, except at home.

(6) Some cases of psychosis or severe emotional disturbance capable of forming relationships with and of accepting help from the speech therapist. It may be pointed out here that the psychosis of some children is not idiopathic but is a reaction to the handicap of severely disordered speech.

(7) The presence of great frustration over the speech difficulty. The awareness of the handicap may be a helpful incentive. Cases which after a long trial prove to be intractable may benefit from the use of gesture.

The speech problems of the mentally deficient child, though varied in nature, have as a basis difficulty in using vocal sound for communication. The child may have no realization of verbal communication beyond the signal level in which case the speech therapist's task consists in helping the child to build from the sound signal level to the level of language as a system of signs and symbols.

Therapeutic methods

(1) The child's experience of failure constitutes a serious problem. There is, among many emotional problems, refusal to persevere. A

straightforward approach is preferable to indiscriminate praise. Once a first difficulty is passed the work may be based on success and the anticipation of achievement. These children, with the exception of those who are emotionally disturbed, may gain benefit from group treatment.

(2) The material chosen should be within the child's grasp and range of interest. Directions should be given in simple words and one stage should be reached before the next command is given, for instance, "Look. Put your tongue up. Say Lah."

(3) Sounds and words should not only be constantly repeated but may also be associated with actions if the child is able to concentrate on both sound and action together. Since the child is able to retain only a limited amount, the first introduction to words should be of immediate practical value, such as family first names, parts of the body, objects used in eating, washing, playing, working and so on. An elementary sentence form which can be applied to many situations may be employed. For example "Put the . . . in the. . . . Put the water in the bowl. Put the soap powder in the bowl. Put the plates in the bowl."

It is advisable to see that one speech skill is mastered before passing on to another. The acquisition and application of elementary sentence forms may have to be taken in two stages. Teachers and parents may help by encouraging the child to use the sentences on suitable occasions. In my opinion pronunciation should be corrected as the words arise in the context.

(4) It is generally believed that backward children lack the power of concentration. Yet many are well able to concentrate, for they are not bored as quickly as more intelligent children and are less easily distracted. However, among the children in training centres there are those who are restive, tire easily or who have some physical weakness. It is as well to start a session with a "news" period, then to intersperse periods of concentration on work with rests. A firm approach is essential and it is helpful to hold a child's head gently in position should he look away.

(6) In treating echolalia it may be helpful to repeat with the child a two-part phrase, with suitable accompanying actions, e.g. "Up and down". The therapist should then stop speaking after saying the

first part of the sentence in order that the child may complete rather than repeat the phrase.

The treatment of children in a training centre is both interesting and rewarding. It is true that practical, scientific and ethical considerations should be taken into account by the speech therapist who is willing to undertake such work. Treatment of a backward child whose response is slow may be at the cost of treatment for two or more intelligent children. It should, however, be remembered that for a mentally deficient child the acquisition or absence of language may mean the difference between being able to work and becoming an increasing burden to the community.

The inability to speak creates great frustration and successful treatment lessens the strain on those who care for the mentally deficient who, when they are able to talk, may become easier to handle. The study of the speech and language of mental deficiency from the scientific viewpoint should also be taken into consideration, for much may be learnt of the processes involved in the acquisition of language, of the nature of linguistic communication and of learning itself through the study of mental deficiency. The knowledge gained can be of practical value in the treatment of intelligent patients. Differing views are expressed about the ethical considerations involved. It should be remembered that these children exist because this community believes it is wrong to deprive them of life and that they have a worth beyond that of intellect. Finally, if there is anything that can be done to relieve suffering, it should be done.

Acknowledgements

I wish to thank the Principal School Medical Officer to the L.C.C., Dr J. A. Scott, for permission to refer to the speech therapy service in training centres and to the pilot scheme.

I should also like to acknowledge the help given to me in this work by Miss Jean Abercrombie, L.C.S.T., who first drew my attention to the importance of speech therapy and general management in the treatment of the training centre child, and the help given by the Hospitaller Brothers of St John of God, through their great interest in the work.

"The machinery underlying the production of sounds and sound combinations in language is very complicated. It consists of a number of parts in addition to the special muscle activity which produces the sound. We know very little about the influence of cortical lesions in all these respects."

Seven years have now elapsed since the second edition of Goldstein's book. Would it not be true to suggest that we still know very little? We might ask if this is because, in general, our ignorance is such that we feel the function of articulation is of such simplicity that little need be said, or whether so little is known that nothing can be said?

The biolinguists Meader and Muyskens (1950) are cautious enough to use the term articulation to mean "merely the production of speech movements, with no implication of 'joining together of sounds' or of syllabification. It involves the muscle movements of larynx, pharynx, and mouth in speech."

It might here be permissible to digress for a moment, to bring this particular field of study to our attention. The two above-mentioned workers regard speech as basically the transformation of biological energy stored up within the organism. Thus it is an integral biological process involving all activities of the body: nutrition, circulation, endocrine activities, etc. The distribution of energy throughout the whole speech mechanism is described as inter-related with the workings of the brain and the development of those organs directly concerned with speech. Thus the findings of anatomists, physicists, neurologists, physiologists, psychologists, economists, sociologists, etc., are all taken into account. "Language is to be regarded as a dynamic, developing group of processes, manifested in the organism (both of the human being and lower animals) and, indeed, constituting an integrated portion of the organism. The organism in its turn is an integrated, functioning portion of its surroundings, including society as a whole and takes on ever new forms through its interactions with the changing forms of its developing environment" (Meader and Muyskens, 1950). The value of such a work as this should not be underestimated, it has a great deal to impart. Nevertheless while I am mainly concerned with our unfortunate tendency to isolate one process of a complex function from another to the point of over-simplification, it would seem to me that here we have a study which reduces the inter-relationships concerned to such a general level as to prevent understanding. One might wonder whether our comprehension of the workings of the human body and mind has really reached such a height, or whether we here find that in an anxiety to have an explanation and a place for everything, several ill-defined concepts and ill-founded hypotheses are constructed.

Let us now look at the definitions of articulation given by those more closely connected with the field of speech therapy.

Van Riper and Irwin (1958) say:

> "Originally, the word articulation referred to the movements of such structures as the lips, jaw and tongue as they modified the flow of voice or air from the larynx. At the present time, articulation also refers to the acoustic impression, to the distinctness or acceptability of the speech sound."

This would suggest that they regard the process as a sensori-motor one, and indeed throughout their work, although they do not appear to say so in so many words, their whole attitude towards articulatory processes indicates that they do not place articulation into a category of pure motor function, as do so many others.

Morley (1959) perhaps places articulation in its rightful place when she says:

> "Articulation is an acquired motor skill developed gradually in early childhood through repeated sensori-motor experience, at conscious and sub-conscious levels, involving constant interplay between the receptor and effector functions."

Later she states:

> "The exact processes by which this function of human behaviour is achieved are still mainly unknown."

It is commonly agreed that we do not know exactly how these processes occur and yet for the purpose of treatment we are forced to make assumptions regarding the disorder which is stated to result from a breakdown in these unknown processes. It is not denied that it is through the study of a breakdown of any activity that insight can be gained, but it is nevertheless wise to remember the extent of our ignorance lest we be tempted to make statements based on insufficient information, and base our diagnostic reasoning on precarious foundations.

We have briefly skimmed over what articulation is thought to be, and we should now consider the beginnings of articulation.

Almost universally it is agreed that the organs of speech are primarily used for other more primitive activities and by the possession of cortical areas for articulation man is enabled to use those organs for the purpose of articulate speech.

It is also generally accepted that babbling plays a part in establishing patterns of articulation for speech though it is not certain exactly how this occurs. Goldstein (1954) while not discounting the value of the babble period states that "its significance in the development of speech is that of acquiring a mastery of muscles which are later going to be concerned in the production of real speech". He maintains that "babbling contains sounds which never appear in later language, which do not exist in the language of the people around the child" and that "the infant loses nearly all the sounds which he has uttered in the babble period". It would be of interest to know whether either of these statements really holds, but it would require a very detailed study to provide us with the answer. If the only purpose of the early babble period were to acquire a mastery of muscles, it might have been just as well achieved by suckling, swallowing, chewing, and other feeding processes. I would suggest that the early babble period is of greater significance inasmuch as those early patterns are used again but not in the same combination of sounds and that, therefore, certain sounds patterns are being laid down which may later be built upon and used in language. They are not lost, unless certain of those sounds are never again required, in which case they may vanish through disuse.

A further interesting though doubtful statement to be found in the works of Goldstein (1954) is that "The first influence from the outer world for language is derived from visual stimulation, and later the control by kinaesthetic and acoustic experience sets in". He gives as an example the earlier fixing of those sounds which can be visually controlled, such as *p*. The acoustic experience he feels, being not for the starting point or control of speaking, but in the finer elaboration of pronunciation.

We might then compare this with the statement of Sapir (1921) that "Language is primarily an auditory system of symbols. Insofar as it is articulated it is also a motor system, but the motor aspect of speech is clearly secondary to the auditory." Whether the early babbling stages are of greater or less importance in the later acquisition of meaningful articulation, or whether visual, acoustic or kinaesthetic senses play the greater part, it would appear that babble has some part to play, and that patterns of articulation are dependent in part upon the sensory system.

Now to consider the problem of dysarthria. Here again one cannot help wondering what is meant by the term dysarthria. Wilfred Trotter (1913) said:

> "Symmetry and the desire for classification are apt to be mistaken for physiological principles and we tend to drift into the error of supposing that conceptions that are clear cut, easily comprehensible and 'reasonable' acquire by that very fact an increased probability of being accurate expositions of the physiological processes they profess to explain. . . ."

It might be well for us to bear this in mind so as not to confuse the explanation of a diagnostic term with that of the disorder referred to.

The term dysarthria literally means disorder of articulation; the term has been reserved for defective articulation due to organic causes. Chief among these causes in childhood are cerebral palsy (including athetosis), cleft palate with or without hare-lip and, less frequently, a defect of development in the nervous system termed "congenital supra-bulbar paresis". According to the terminology of the College of Speech Therapists it is a neuro-muscular articulatory disorder in which the muscle tone as well as reflex actions such as swallowing, suckling and chewing are usually affected. It is manifest in slurred, weak, laboured, explosive and other forms of distorted articulation and also incoordinated phonation and respiration. (No distinction is here made between anarthria and dysarthria.)

Penfield (1958) defines anarthria and dysarthria as "a difficulty in the articulation of words. This may include the motor employment of muscles of respiration and vocalization as well as lips, tongue and throat." This "motor phenomenon . . . may be produced by a lesion in the motor face-area situated in the cortex of either hemisphere". He uses anarthria and dysarthria interchangeably apparently to describe the degree of difficulty in using the mouth and tongue and throat for the purposes of speaking. Since Penfield certainly regards dysarthria as a motor disorder one might suggest that a very fine line is being drawn to place this disorder entirely into the area of motor function. Earlier in his book he regards the motor area of the cortex as an arrival platform and departure platform the purpose of which is to transmute the patterned stream of impulses arriving from the centrencephalic system and to transmit them to the voluntary muscles.

Morley (1959) mentions "abnormality of movement of the muscles for articulation with abnormal reflex activity and muscle tone" in dysarthria, but also stresses that "the receptor system is normal but can only act through a damaged effector mechanism". She draws attention to a possible over-simplification in the classifications given. Again there is the implication of a fine line being drawn between the receptor and effector mechanisms.

The above-mentioned definitions rest on the tacit assumption that in the cases covered the neurological findings suggest a normal receptor mechanism. This is not the place to discuss the means of approach by which this may be ascertained. For the sake of argument it may be asked, however, is it possible to ascertain whether the receptor mechanism is normal? Certain empirical findings met in treatment seem to indicate that in cases of lower motor neurone lesions it may well be that the receptor system is normal. In cases due to lesions of the upper motor neurone system we have, I submit, reasons to think that this is not the case.

Since we do not know exactly how, by a lesion, the function of the brain is modified in such a way as to produce dysarthria, we can only make certain assumptions which we must be prepared to change or modify continually in the light of new findings. Walsh (1948), in criticizing modern thought on the motor cortex and the pyramidal tract, says "It has considered both in so complete an isolation from the rest of the nervous system, that the essential importance of the sensory side of that system has been forgotten". To attempt, therefore, to divide the sensory from the motor system seems to me to be inviting difficulties in deciding on the rationale of the treatment of dysarthria.

Treatment

For the purpose of discussing the therapeutic approach the dysarthrias may be divided into those resultant from an upper motor neurone lesion and those resultant from a lower motor neurone lesion.

Methods of treatment, while varying to some degree, fall into two main categories: (1) specific exercises for the movements of the lip, tongue, palate and jaw, together with breathing exercises, and (2) the motor-kinaesthetic method.

A number of authors recommend exercises for the palate which include: blowing, yawning, panting, gargling, repeated swallowing; for the jaw: opening and shutting of the mouth, deliberate protrusion and retrusion of the jaw, lateral and rotary movements; for the lips: flexion and extension of the lips, repeating with force the sounds, *p, b, m, w, f* and *v*, protrusion of upper and then lower lip, creating of intra-oral tension against compressed lips; for the tongue: protrusion movements up and down, from side to side while protruded, the practice of all consonants. Since, as we have earlier mentioned in the terminology, respiration and phonation are often affected, vocal and breathing exercises of varying types are recommended, most of which require a high degree of coordination.

Froeschels (1943) advocates particularly jaw shaking from side to side and his "chewing method", requiring the opening and closing of the mouth, flexing and extending of the tongue with simultaneous vocalization.

Many therapists place importance on visual stimulation and have their patients watch both the therapist and themselves in a mirror. Opinions vary on the value of auditory training in the treatment of dysarthria but it seems that ear-training is frequently used. Tactile stimulation is also mentioned in some works: the patient is taught where to put his lips, tongue and jaw. He feels, by the relationship of the one to the other, the positions of the organs of speech.

It is agreed that such methods are of value, should the dysarthria occur as a result of a lower motor neurone lesion, producing a weakness of the muscles. It is then a question of strengthening weak muscles, or attempting to strengthen them by exercise, or to find a means of compensating for a definite paralysis of certain parts of the musculature.

In cases of upper motor neurone disorder, however, an attempt to train or retrain the musculature by specific exercises would appear to be an unwise and rather fruitless procedure. The musculature of a patient suffering from an upper motor neurone disorder is not weak or paralysed, the muscle tone is abnormal; this in its turn leads to an unbalancing of movement. Even if the exercises described above seem in the end to achieve some success it will have been with great effort and struggle on the part of the patient and it is doubtful whether the success will be maintained, since it will be imposing a good pattern upon a bad one by strengthening that which is not weak, but incoordinated.

The second method, that is, the motor-kinaesthetic method, was first described in great detail by Edna Hill Young, about thirty years ago in a private communication, and recommended for use in all defects of articulation. She said, "the motor-kinaesthetic method guides the muscles from one unit into the connecting movement or preparation process for the next sound production unit". In exemplifying the procedure, Edna Hill Young says:

> "I want the child to say 'foot'. I take the lower lip and bring it upward against the upper incisors, doing the same with my own mouth, and moving the air outward. As soon as this voiceless sound is heard, and as a preparatory movement for the next sound, I immediately move the lips outward and slightly toward the centre, so that the vowel position is sensed in normal timing."

Her aim in using this method in the treatment of the cerebral palsied person, was that "movements should be habituated correctly when first gained, or neuro-muscular difficulties may later develop through changes in movement needed for correction".

This method was also, to some extent, used by Peacher (1947) in the treatment of patients suffering from dysarthria following war injuries. Later still it was developed by Pauline Marland together with Dr and Mrs Karel Bobath (1959) in the treatment of the cerebral palsied. Marland and Bobath, working together, developed the idea that since posture was necessary for all activities, the treatment of dysarthria in the cerebral palsied should be carried out with the patient in a position in which the abnormal reflex movements were inhibited. This because, as Bobath writes "Normal muscle tone is necessary for the performance of normal movements. Muscle tone should be steady and of moderate intensity if performance is to be smooth and precise." This form of treatment brought about a close link between speech therapy and physiotherapy.

We know that in the early stages of normal development movements are primitive and widespread; as the higher areas of the brain take over control, these widespread primitive movements are, to some extent, inhibited and modified in order to allow more selective and purposeful movements to take place. Whether one is referring to the movements of the hand or of the tongue, this developmental process is the same. If, owing to a lesion, the higher areas do not take over, then these widespread primitive movements are not inhibited, and the selective movements are unable to take place.

Thus in the method used by those who work with the Bobaths the abnormal movements are first inhibited and then normal movements are facilitated; the speech therapist gives the patient, as far as is possible, the sensation of the normal pattern in breathing, vocalization and articulation. She makes use of the auditory sensations by repeating the sound so that the patient may hear it; if necessary, the visual sense is used by having the patient in a position in which he may see the therapist's mouth. In this method babbling is used, not only in individual sounds but in sequences of sounds, and the sounds are so facilitated as to produce words as quickly as possible, since it is believed that it is important to lay down patterns of normal articulation from the outset.

So far we have mentioned dysarthria only from the articulatory point of view, but it should be remembered that there is frequently a language difficulty too. It is rare to find a dysarthria resulting from an upper motor neurone disorder without an accompanying degree of dysphasia or of apparent dysphasia. It is debatable that this may be due to the fact that since, in these cases, sounds are incorrectly produced, the word patterns are also incorrect and therefore there is an incorrect feed-back of the kinaesthetic sensation.

In cases of so-called "isolated dysarthria" met in cases of congenital supra-bulbar paresis, I have yet to see a case without an exceedingly delayed language development. As an example, here are descriptions of a picture, given by children who had been diagnosed as suffering from congenital supra-bulbar paresis. Both children are 10 years of age and are describing a picture of a toy-shop.

> 1st child: "A boy and a little girl – and a father. Father looks at train, and the – little boy looks at Teddy Bear."
>
> 2nd child: "The man takes his children to a – toyshop. The children looking at toys. See car, big car. Girl sees dog's bath, she buyed – (a long pause as though she knew this wasn't right) – buyed it. They are looking at a – what do you call it? – a Teddy Bear."

I have frequently heard similar difficulties in such cases and I would suggest that it should seriously be considered whether the diagnosis "isolated dysarthria" is warranted.

In conclusion I should like to say that while I have suggested that dysarthria is not a purely motor disorder, I have made an attempt to re-draw attention to the fact that one cannot isolate the motor from the sensory, and that an involvement of the one is bound to involve, to a greater or lesser extent, the other; that there is a danger of over-simplification and that this simplicity tends to under-estimate the damage and ultimately affect treatment.

REFERENCES

Bobath, K. (1959) "Neuropathology of Cerebral Palsy and its Importance in Treatment and Diagnosis", *C.P. Bulletin* **1**, No. 8, pp. 13–33

Froeschels, E. (1943) "A Contribution to the Pathology and Therapy of Dysarthria due to certain Cerebral Lesions", *Journal of Speech Disorders* **8**, 301

Goldstein, K. (1954) *Language and Language Disturbances*, New York, Greene & Stratton

Hill-Young, E. Signed Communication, entitled "Directed Speech Help for the Cerebral Palsied"

Meader, C. L., and Muyskens, G. H. (1950) *Handbook of Biolinguistics* Part I, Section A, London, Pitman
Morley, M. E. (1959) "Defects of Articulation", *Folia Phon.* **11**, Nos. 1–3
Peacher, W. G. (1947) "Speech Disorders in World War II", *J. Nerv and Ment. Dis.* 106/1
Penfield, W., and Roberts, L. (1959) *Speech and Brain Mechanisms*, Oxford University Press
Sapir, E. (1921) *Language*, London, C.U.P.
Terminology for Speech Pathology (1959), College of Speech Therapists
Trotter, W. (1913) *J. Psychol. u. Neurol.* **20**, Ergänzungsheft, 2, 102
Van Riper, and Irwin, G. V. (1958) *Voice and Articulation*, New Jersey, Prentice Hall
Walsh, F. M. R.. (1948) *Critical Studies in Neurology*, Edinburgh, Livingstone
Ziman, John (1960) "Science is Social", the *Listener*, August

21

OLIVÉ DUFFIE, London

A Pilot Scheme for Speech Therapy in Training Centres

The purpose of the pilot scheme was to see how – to what extent and in what way – mentally deficient children, ineducable even in schools for the educationally sub-normal but able to benefit from special training in day centres, could be helped by speech therapy. The range of intelligence quotient is from 49 to 25, most of the children having an intelligence quotient between 45 and 33. After the experimental year a regular service was extended to all the junior centres (with a total of over five hundred children). It has thus been possible to follow the progress of some of the children over a four-year period.

The main aims were to find: (1) Criteria for use in the selection of patients able to benefit. (2) Therapeutic methods to suit their special needs. (3) Specific methods and general management to stimulate speech and language.

In my opinion most of these children need specially designed methods of approach to their speech both at home and in the centres. This alone is not enough; selected cases can benefit by speech therapy. Those who received regular treatment showed progress, while others showed much less, or no progress.

Of seventy children seen during a first survey: (1) 20% had no speech, (2) 40% had very defective speech, (3) 10% had serviceable speech though with minor defects, (4) 20% were slowly developing speech, (5) 10% had normal speech. These figures are approximate.

The terms normal and defective speech are used here to mean respectively "speech correct as to articulation and grammatical structure" and "speech deviating from this standard" – in both

CATHERINE E. RENFREW, Oxford

Speech Therapy with Backward Children

In his book *Speech and the Development of Mental Processes in the Child*, the Russian psychologist Luria (1959) has described the study of identical twins whose speech was severely retarded since they used only a small number of barely differentiated sounds. The twins behaved in a lively, competent manner and were later found to be of average intelligence, yet their play was monotonous and they showed no ability to construct or use play material imaginatively. They displayed no interest in drawing or modelling. At the first examination, which took place when they were five years old, it was found that they did not understand completely what was said to them, nor did they listen to stories read to them, although their hearing was normal. The twins were separated and placed in different groups in a kindergarten in order that objective assessments of the development of speech could be made. During this time, one twin, the weaker, was given special help with his speech. Shortly after separation it was found that the speech of both twins showed positive development and had reached normal standards within ten months. Their mental development during this period was also marked. Their play showed imagination and greater variety, they were able to solve problems, construct objects and formulate aims for their activity. The twin who had special help with his speech greatly surpassed his brother in language development, using grammatically constructed and extended sentences at an earlier stage. He became the more active in planning a project and showed initiative in carrying it through; he also showed himself capable of more rational thinking. In other respects, for instance in motor activity, the untrained twin still maintained the lead. This experiment may demonstrate how closely linked the speech process can be with mental development. It may also illustrate that it is possible for children to make fuller use of and develop their innate mental capacity.

If we accept that speech and mental development are closely related, it seems to me that in the education of the mentally handicapped stress should be laid on the development of the understanding and use of speech. Acting on this premise I have considerably altered my role as speech therapist in a school for educationally subnormal (E.S.N.) children during the last four years.

I work for two three-hour sessions a week in a school for 120 E.S.N. children aged from five to sixteen. Most of the children have I.Q's ranging from 50–75, and are transferred to the E.S.N. school when about seven years old. I test the speech of all entrants, assessing four aspects: (1) articulation, (2) auditory memory – nonsense syllables and sentences, (3) vocabulary, (4) sentence formulation. I use these tests as a basis for comparison of improvement from year to year. Any child who is more retarded on these speech tests than his mental age warrants receives so-called "conventional speech therapy" on which I spend three hours a week. During the other three hours I do group and class work dealing with every child in the school until he is ten years old. I also do special group work with seven selected inarticulate children who are over ten years old. All this group and class work is done in closest cooperation with the teacher, for it is our joint concern that these children should, through the medium of developing language, be influenced in their modes of learning.

The teacher's first task is to attract the children's attention so that they will listen and respond to speech. Observation shows that these children are generally inattentive unless they are startled by an unexpected tone of voice. It is noticeable that the teacher supplements speech with gesture. This gesturing, at first necessary to convey meaning, becomes habitual in the teacher's behaviour, and it is accepted from the children. The speech therapist may help these children, without gesture, to attend to speech.

With the youngest children I am mainly concerned with the development of speech in social situations. The children take part in specially devised social experiences, hearing the customary speech accompaniment. The family at home, food, toys and pets are the main topics that produce response from the children. The temptation, of course, is for the therapist to talk too much, to be unable to tolerate a gap and therefore to get no response because she is too stimulating. Shopping is another useful activity which serves various purposes. The children have to be taught how to ask for goods – at first they are likely to hand the money to the shopkeeper without realizing that words are needed. They apparently do not realize that they can manipulate their environment by the use of words. Real shopping can be overwhelming for many of the children and it is replaced by a term of toy shopping in the staffroom. The names of objects are learned as they are handled. Then the actual buying and selling is played, when possible, with the goods out of sight so that an effort is made to remember the names. All this makes the necessary repetition meaningful, and the words being used in different contexts often enables a concept of the meaning to be formed. In this way a non-verbal signal (coin) is gradually superseded by a verbal one which in due course becomes a sign (name of the object).

Verbal disagreements may be encouraged, for in this way conversation between children arises normally and sometimes elementary reasoning will take place. If feeling can be verbalized it is more accessible to modification, which is a form of learning.

Two uses of language are to facilitate thought and assist memory. So vocabulary is built by the use of pictures and objects, by imitation of words, by the identification of words in answer to questions and to questions that give no visual clue.

The questions mentally handicapped children ask tend to be repetitious, taking the form of attention-seeking chatter. They evince little curiosity, possibly due to the fact that they are slow in seeing relationships. I work with two groups of inarticulate boys over ten. Although their I.Q's, except for one spastic boy, are among the highest in the school, they are all excessively shy and lacking in confidence. We play games of the "twenty questions" variety, and they have all responded to this mental training. It would appear, therefore, that here again statements decoded by us as information seeking are used as signals inducing us to establish and maintain contact.

The speech therapist's approach to formal preparation for reading takes various forms which may not be used by the class teacher. Accurate repetition of sentences of increasing length help to extend the desirable auditory memory. Practice in speaking sentences is usually desirable before learning to read.

In my opinion the function of the speech therapist working with mentally handicapped children is twofold: to assist the child to extend his experience and to help him acquire language in which he can think and talk about such experience. I feel sure we could as a profession make a contribution in this field and perhaps elucidate something of the nature of the relationship between speech and mental development.

REFERENCE

Luria, A. R. (1959) *Speech and the Development of Mental Processes in the Child*, London, Staples Press

23

D. E. COLLINS, Ashtead

Some Problems Facing the Adult with Progressive Deafness, and Lipreading

The reception of spoken thought by the adult who is becoming deaf must take place through the eyes as well as the ears, and the degree of reception through the eyes varies according to the amount of residual hearing or the amount which can be conveyed by a hearing aid.

The ability to learn to lipread is not confined to those of younger years or the better educated, but is more closely connected first with personality – the man or woman who is perhaps more of an extrovert, who is determined not to lose contact with the world of normal hearing and who realizes that help comes primarily from within himself. The incentive to acquire a new code of signals and signs is connected with necessity, for example where perhaps a job may be lost because of increasing deafness.

Many elderly and old people learn to lipread amazingly quickly – perhaps because they have learnt to be patient, are not over-anxious and generally have a relatively calm outlook on life. They, like some younger people, are often hampered by poor eyesight.

Since many teachers of the deaf are not prepared to teach lipreading to adults who are going deaf, it may often be the speech therapist who is called upon to help.

There are three main considerations to bear in mind when approaching the subject of teaching lipreading:

1. The social position in which the adult faced with progressive deafness finds himself.

2. The difficulty the speech therapist may meet in concentrating on what speech *looks like*, because the very nature of her work has made her concentrate more on listening to speech and feeling speech.

3. The teacher of lipreading must have a sensitive and fertile imagination when she plans her lessons and teaching material.

Despite the fact that there is now more knowledge of deafness among the general public through the media of television, radio and films, the deaf person is still probably one of the most misunderstood in the world. It is, I think, significant of man's inability to understand the disability of deafness that throughout the history of drama blindness has frequently played an important part in tragedy but deafness has been only a minor comic.

The deaf person feeling he is a nuisance tends to avoid human society. His deafness comes between him and his fellows like an impenetrable wall and he is often lonely, gloomy, listless and discouraged. This depressive attitude is reflected on the therapist who then finds it sometimes difficult to help. Many are ashamed of their deafness and this accounts for the fact that those who would find a hearing aid a great help, often refuse to wear one. Quite mistakenly, they fear that by wearing an aid and so advertising their deafness they may lose their jobs, their friends and their social contacts. Those who are born deaf tend to mix almost entirely with their fellow deaf. This is partly the result of education in special schools from which they move quite naturally on to the Clubs for the Deaf. The adult who is going deaf feels he fits neither into the world of the deaf nor into that of the hearing. He needs to be helped to remain in the hearing world. (The born deaf, too, needs to be helped to move out of his rather confined circle into the hearing world.)

To teach lipreading successfully it is a great help to be able to *feel* as far as possible as the pupil feels. Once he realizes his predicament is known and understood he will respond to teaching in a way which is encouraging both to himself and the teacher.

The teacher of lipreading must concentrate on what speech *looks like* when it cannot be heard, a task which is, at first, by no means easy. The teacher must learn to see speech as a series of moving pictures – pictures which may be single shapes, that is, a vowel or consonant, single words, or words grouped in phrases or sentences, or whole paragraphs and passages. It must also be remembered that, although the speech of two people living in the same district with a similar background may sound alike, no two people look alike when they are speaking. The basic movements or shapes are, of course, similar; for instance, the coming together and parting of the lips for P, B and M (which, incidentally, illustrates one of the great difficulties speech presents to the lipreader: certain sounds appear to be identical in their formation although they sound quite different from each other. One speaker may have full mobile lips, and one may have thin lips, one may speak with the minimum of jaw movements and one may over-articulate, thinking that by so doing he will help the lipreader, whereas in fact he is distorting the visual aspect of the speech signs.)

Facial expression is a great help to real understanding, and the person who uses his eyes and face to add colour, as it were, to his speech is much easier to lipread than his more expressionless companion. The speech therapist who contemplates teaching lipreading should habituate herself to observing people's facial expression whenever possible: What can we learn of them by their expressions? How do they use their faces when they converse? It is well to remember that intonation, stress, and accent are lost with increasing deafness – facial expression can compensate to some extent for these prosodemes. To take an example, intonation rises towards the end of a question – and almost always the eyebrows move upwards when a question is asked. This is a simple but valuable clue for the lipreader.

The third and final point which is closely allied to the first two is the necessity of having a sensitive and fertile imagination when planning lipreading lessons. Two considerations have been taken into account in the selection of material. First, it has to be suitable and of interest to the pupil or group. When teaching a group this may be difficult because it may comprise people of varying ages and from different walks of life. For instance, one group consisted of two retired clergymen, a young Civil Service clerk, two elderly retired ladies who lived a solitary life in a small guest house, two middle-aged housewives and an old man who had been a manual worker on the railways all his life. In this particular group it was the old railway worker who learned most quickly! Intellect and education thus have little bearing on the ability to learn lipreading.

Individual pupils cannot be taught successfully if the identical lesson is given for each one. There must, of course, be a basic plan but this should be flexible. The first lessons consist of building up a picture alphabet in order that the deafened adult may quickly recognize the shapes and movements of speech sounds. More general exercises need adaptation for different people. This means much work for the teacher and is a challenge to her versatility.

The second consideration is the usefulness of the material in order to illustrate the theory of lipreading. Words, phrases, sentences and paragraphs are selected as examples of specific speech images or pictures.

Lipreading is a combination of the ability to lipread accurately those things which cannot be guessed, and the ability to observe and size up a situation in order to know almost before the speaker opens his mouth what he is going to say. Many deafened adults gain these abilities, some in a remarkably short time.

To me, teaching lipreading is fascinating, interesting and always rewarding. I know that in teaching it I have added to my knowledge in many ways and that I have increased my own powers of expression. I am grateful to my many pupils who, knowing they are moving into ever-increasing silence, have taught *me* much, have helped me to understand their difficulties and problems and have shown me the true value of patient and determined courage.

INDEX

Abercrombie, J., 200
Adrian, E. D., 12, 18
Agrammatism, 39, 40
Aids to diagnosis, 83–86, 93–100
Alalia, 99
Aldridge, C. H., 93
Allbright, J. S. and R. W., 38, 43
Allomorph, 34
Allophone, 20, 26, 27, 28, 33, 153, 155, 158, 163
Allophoneme, 28
Anarthria, 188
Anima, 106
Animus, 103
Anthropologist, work of, 9, 11, 134
Anxiety neurosis, 99
Anxiety symptom, 112
Aphasia, 39, 40, 58, 99, 166–174
Aphonia, 167
Archephoneme, 16, 17
Aristotle, 17, 160
Arkhipoua, O. G., 100
Arnold, G. E., 37, 43, 177, 178, 182
Articulatory disorder, 131
Ashley-Montagu, R. F., 15
Ataxia, 108
Athetosis, 188
Audio-analyser, 83, 85
Audiometer, 84
Averbukh, I. S., 100

Bartlett, F. C., 57
Batten, L., 166, 174
Beecher, H. W., 6
Berkeley, G., 15
Biologist, work of, 11 ff.

Birmingham, Bishop of, xi, 1
Bloomfield, L., 21, 22, 42
Bobath, K., 191, 192, 193
Borel-Maisonny, S., 43
Born, M., 62 ff., 64
Brain, W. R., 57, 173, 174
Brook, F., 95, 100
Brook, J. R., 83
Brough, J., 18
Butfield, E., 43

Cantor, G., 57
Carroll, J. B., 10, 18
Carter, P., 101
Cerebellar defect, 108
Cerebral palsy, 188, 191, 192
Chromatrope, 55, 63, 64
Cicero, 5
Cleft palate, 188
 speech, 163
Clutter, 91, 172, 177, 178, 180
College of Speech Therapists, *see* Terminology
Collins, D. E., 205
Communication Theory, x, 12, 15
Commutation, 23
Congenital supra-bulbar paresis, 183, 193
Contrastive substitution, 23
Critchley, M., 159, 165, 171, 173, 174

Dalton, J., 54
Davie, M. R., 140
Deafness, 108, 205–208
Dementia, 169

INDEX

Distinctive features, 24 ff., 42, 153
Distinctive sounds, 24 ff.
Douglas, M., 134, 139
Drawings, in therapy, 117–129, 134–136
Dubois, R. J., 17, 18
Duffie, O., 195
Dysarthria, 99, 108, 161, 162, 171, 177, 183–193, 196, 198
Dyslalia, 36 ff., 49, 86, 121, 131, 139, 141–165, 177
Dysphasia, 49, 171, 192, 198
Dysphonia, 91, 198
Dyspraxia, 171, 177, 198

Echolalia, 199
Eclampsia, 178
Einstein, A., 62 ff., 64
Eisler, Goldman-, F., 68 ff.
Ellis, M. J., 109
Epstein, A. G., 131, 139, 164, 165

Feedback, 40, 70
Ferreira, A. J., 138, 139
Firth, J. R., 42
Fisher, J., 143, 151, 165
Fitch, D. B., 175
Florenskaya, V. A., 100
Fordham, M., 116, 130
Formant theory, 79
Frank, J., 160, 165
Fraser, F. R., 12, 18
Free variant, 28
Frued, S., 15
Froeschels, E., 190, 193
Fry, D. B., xi, 35, 43, 65, 85

Gardiner, A., vii, 13
Gaynor, F., 158
Glossectomy, 39
Glottal stop, 110, 112, 113, 114, 115
Goldstein, K., 184, 187, 193
Grady, P. A. E., 159
Greene, M., 43
Grewel, F., 42, 43

Grimm, J., 33
Guthrie, D., 131, 139

Haas, W., xi, 9, 18, 20, 34, 165
Halle, M., 158
Hare-lip, 188
Harris, Z. S., 18, 150, 151, 152, 153, 158
Hartley, L. M., 152
Head, H., 57
Hearing loss, *see* deafness
Hebb, D. O., 57
Hesitation phenomena, 68
Hemiplegia, 168
Hill-Young, E., 191, 193
Hippocrates, 160
Hjelmslev, L., 23
Hockett, C. F., 10, 18, 158, 163, 165
Howe, G., 116
Howell, J., x
Hyper-rhinophonia, 38
Hypo-rhinophonia, 38
Hysteria, 99

Idiolect, 133
Information theory, 68
Innes, M., xii
Irwin, G. V., 186, 194

Jackson, J. H., 11, 18, 110, 113, 115, 116
Jakobson, R., 16, 18, 42, 156, 158
Jespersen, O., 131, 139
Johnson, S., 50, 61
Jung, C. G., 15, 16, 18, 130
Jungian theory, 103

Kainz, F., 43
Kander, G., 43
Keller, A. G., 140
Kerényi, C., 130
Kluckhohn, C., 12, 18

Language, quantum of, 50–64
Laryngectomy, 39

INDEX

Lenneburg, E. H., 36, 42
Lévi-Strauss, C., 10, 12, 18
Lewis, M. M., 131, 132, 139
Linguist, work of, 9 ff.
Linguistics, historical, 44-49
Linguistics, relation to speech pathology, 33-42, 144-165
Lipreading, 205-208
Logopedics, 35, 87 ff.
Logoscope, 93-100
Lower motor neurone lesion, 189, 190
Lubbock, J., 11, 18
Luchsinger, R., 37, 43
Luria, A. R., 61, 201

Marland, P., 40, 43, 191
Martinet, A., xi, 16, 18
Mason, S. E., xii, 131
Mayo, B., 15, 18
Meader, C. L., 185, 194
Meredith, G. P., xi, 50
Mol, H., 88, 92
Möller-Nielsen, E., 145, 151
Mongol, 85, 198
Morley, M. E., 43, 142 ff., 151, 186, 188, 194
Morpheme, 17, 34, 40, 67, 68, 80, 81 ff.
Muyskens, G. H., 185, 194

Nash, F. A., 93 ff., 99, 100
Negus, V. E., 112, 116
Nessel, E., 40, 43
Neumann, E., 133, 139
Newton, I., 64

Ockham, W., 56
Oldfield, R. C., 57
Orton, S. T., 116
Oscillograph, 74
Oscilloscope, 83, 85

Palatal defects, 91
Paradigm, 23

Paranoia, 99
Pararhesis, 139
Parker, L. P., 183
Partridge, E., 134, 139
Peacher, W. G., 191, 194
Pei, M. A., 158
Penfield, W., 36, 184, 188 ff., 194
Phenylketonuria, 86
Phone, 153, 154, 157, 163
Phoneme, 17, 20, 26, 27, 28, 30, 31, 33, 34, 67, 68, 70, 71, 77, 80, 81, 82, 153 ff., 162, 163, 179, 182
Phonemic analysis, 16, 144, 150, 153
Phonotactic features, 31
Pike, K., 157, 158, 164, 165
Plato, 16, 17
Pollitt, J., 117
Prosodic features, 31
Psychologist, work of, 10
Psychosis, 197, 198

Redundancy, role of, 80 ff., 157
Reichenbach, H., 63
Religion, as therapy, 2 ff.
Renfrew, C. E., 163, 165, 201
Rhema, 17, 139
Rhematologist, work of, 17 ff.
Rhematology, 17
Rhememe, 17
Rhotacism, 142, 179
Ritchie, D., 169, 174
Roberts, L., 36, 194
Ross, A. S. C., xi, 44
Ruesch, J., 12, 18
Ryle, G., 52

Sapir, E., 16, 18, 188, 194
Saussure, F. de, 21
Seth, G., 131, 139
Shames, G., 143, 151, 164, 165
Sigmatism, 142, 179
Signal, 101, 102, 103, 106, 108, 116, 131, 134, 135

INDEX

Signal, linguistic, x, 7, 12, 13, 15, 16, 20–32, 55, 56, 58, 63, 66, 72 ff., 80, 90, 91, 109, 113, 132, 137, 138, 157, 198, 203, 205
Sign, linguistic, x, 7, 12, 15, 16, 20, 22, 109, 132, 137, 138, 198, 203, 205
  in diagnosis, 93, 113, 116, 131, 161
Simms, R. E., 141
Snow, C. P., 52
Sociologist, work of, 10 ff.
Sound level meter, 85
Spectograph, 74, 85
Speech, coding and decoding, 65–82
"Speech therapists", work of, 14 ff.
"Speech therapy", place among sciences, 7–19
Spencer, H., 102
Stammer, ix, 8, 40, 91, 95–99, 101–108, 115, 120, 124, 127, 129, 160, 173, 176, 198
Steer, M. D., 88, 92, 95
Stein, L., xii, 2, 7, 11, 12, 16, 19, 44, 83, 100, 110, 112, 113, 115, 116, 131, 137, 139, 165, 168
Steinthal, H., 131, 139
Stroboscope, 85
Sumner, H. G., 134, 139
Sutherland, J., 6
Symbol, linguistic, x, 7, 15, 29, 91, 109, 132, 137, 138, 163, 167, 188, 198
  psychological, 13 ff., 16, 116, 118, 120, 125, 129, 134, 135

Syntagmeme, 17
Synthetic Speech, 75

Tape recorders, 83
Taxeme, 40
Teacher of languages, work of, 10
Terminology, of College of Speech Therapists, 37, 131, 161, 166, 188
Throat microphone, 84
Training Centres, pilot scheme in, 195–200
Trim, J. L. M., xi, 33, 165
Trotter, W., 188, 194
Trubetzkoy, N. S., 16, 19

Upper motor neurone lesion, 189, 190 ff., 192

Valentine, C. W., 116
Van Riper, C., 99, 131, 140, 164, 165, 186, 194
Van Thal, J. H., 87, 161, 165
Vernon, M., 57

Walsh, F. M. R., 189, 194
Weekley, E., 13, 19
Wickes, F., 130
Wilkins, J. L., 166
Wilson, J. L., *see* Birmingham, Bishop of
Wittgenstein, L., 54
Wolters, A. W. P., 57
Word-frame, function, 23

Zangwill, O. L., 57
Ziman, J., 183, 194